DETERMINANTS OF EXPENDITURES FOR PHYSICIANS' SERVICES IN THE UNITED STATES 1948-68

VICTOR R. FUCHS
City University of New York
Mount Sinai School of Medicine
National Bureau of Economic Research

MARCIA J. KRAMER
National Bureau of Economic Research

NATIONAL CENTER FOR HEALTH SERVICES RESEARCH AND DEVELOPMENT

DHEW Publication No. (HSM) 73-3013
Department of Health, Education and Welfare
Health Services and Mental Health Administration
December 1972

**National Bureau
of Economic Research**

OCCASIONAL PAPER 117

Library of Congress card number: 74-188339
ISBN number: 0-87014-247-X
Printed in the United States of America

PREFACE

This paper was prepared at the National Bureau of Economic Research at the request of and with financial assistance provided by the National Center for Health Services Research and Development, U.S. Department of Health, Education, and Welfare.

Our principal objective is to gain a better understanding of the factors that determine expenditures for physicians' services in the United States. We attempt to do this through analyses of trends over time and of variations across states at a given point in time. The statistical decomposition of the time series was largely the work of Fuchs, while Kramer assumed primary responsibility for the econometric cross-section analysis. The complete paper, however, represents a collaborative effort for which both authors take full responsibility.

We are indebted to Barry Chiswick, Martin Feldstein, Michael Grossman, Anne Scitovsky, Christopher Sims, Finis Welch, Robert Willis, and three anonymous National Center reviewers for their constructive comments and suggestions. We are also grateful to Atherton Bean, Charles Berry, and Emilio Collado, NBER directors who provided helpful comments. For their highly valued research assistance, we extend thanks to Carol Breckner, Phyllis Goldberg, and Robert Linn. We are grateful to Terry Battipaglia and Maria Perides for preparation of the manuscript, to Hedy D. Jellinek for her editorial services, and to H. Irving Forman for the figures and charts.

Extensive use is made of the results of surveys conducted by *Medical Economics*, and we wish to express our appreciation to the editors of that journal for their cooperation. Finally, we should like to acknowledge the valuable assistance of the following members of the NBER Health Economics Advisory Committee: Morton D. Bogdonoff, M.D.; James Brindle; Norton Brown, M.D.; Kurt Deuschle, M.D. (chairman); Marion B. Folsom; Eli Ginzberg; the late George James, M.D.; Richard Kessler, M.D.; and the late David Lyall, M.D.

Victor R. Fuchs

Marcia J. Kramer

ACKNOWLEDGMENT

This monograph, one of three publications* commissioned by the Publications Advisory Board of the National Center for Health Services Research and Development (NCHSRD), was prepared under contract with the authors. The opinions expressed are those of the authors and do not necessarily reflect the official position of the NCHSRD, its administrative parent Health Services and Mental Health Administration, or any other agency of the U.S. Government.

PAB Membership:

Dr. Bernard G. Greenberg (CHAIRMAN)
Mr. Robert E. Toomey
Dr. Howard E. Freeman
Dr. Robert J. Haggerty
Prof. Herbert E. Klarman, Ph.D.

Mrs. Anne Scitovsky
Dr. Rosemary Stevens
Dr. Ralph Straetz
Dr. Charles R. Wright
Mr. Domenic A. Fuccillo, Jr. (Secretary)

*The two others are: Martin Feldstein, *Rising Cost of Hospital Care;* and Ralph Straetz and Marvin Lieberman (eds.), *Decision Making and Control.*

CONTENTS

TABLES

CHARTS

FIGURES

Introduction and Summary

Introduction

Expenditures for physicians' services in the United States increased by 328 per cent between 1948 and 1969—a growth rate considerably more rapid than that of gross national product or personal consumption expenditures, and about the same as that of other services.[1] This paper examines the rise in expenditures for physicians' services and attempts to explain the pattern of change in the decades following World War II. We also analyze the very large geographical differences in expenditures per capita that exist in the United States. Our study should contribute to an understanding of the economics of medical care and to an improvement in the nation's ability to predict and control such expenditures in the future.

Concern over the cost of medical care is widespread. Special attention has been focused on the rapid rise in the price of and the expenditures for physicians' services because it is said that these services are essential, that the price is not determined in a competitive market, and that consumer ignorance gives the physician unusual control over the quantity and type of service provided. Furthermore, the extensive growth of third-party payment, through both private insurance and governmental programs, is believed to exacerbate inflationary pressures in this area by reducing the net price to the consumer and thus encouraging utilization.

The essentiality argument is a complex one and rests as much on subjective beliefs as on objective evidence. Basically, a service can be considered essential on two grounds. The first applies where the demand for the service is relatively insensitive to changes in income—where it is regarded as so necessary that (in the absence of philanthropy, sliding fee scales, or third-party payment) families with low incomes devote a relatively large portion of their budget to it. Some elements of physicians' services are clearly necessities in this sense, e.g., surgery for an inflamed appendix. Many physicians' services, however, ranging from well-baby care through annual checkups to elective surgery, are not so clearly necessities, while still others (like cosmetic surgery) might well be classed as luxuries.

A second criterion of essentiality applies to a service the consumption of which involves important external effects. Thus, basic education for all is considered essential in the United States partly because of the belief that the failure to educate some will have serious unfavorable repercussions on others. A similar argument concerning physicians' services could be advanced with respect to treatment of communicable diseases. At one time such diseases occupied the bulk of physicians' time, but currently they are much less important.

Probably more important than the essentiality argument is the peculiar nature of the market for physicians' services. When a good or service (without significant external effects in either production or consumption) is produced and sold under reasonably competitive conditions, there is usually no special need for public attention or public policy. In such cases, changes in price and expenditures presumably reflect the true cost to society of producing the good or service and the knowledgeable judgment of consumers regarding its value. With respect to physicians' services, the imperfections of competition are numerous and powerful. On the supply side, these include the restrictions on entry created by licensure and professional control of medical education, the limitations on practice implicit in the hospital appointment system, and the absence of price cutting, advertising, and other forms of rivalry. As for demand, the difficulty consumers experience in judging the quality of physicians' services is well known, and it is thought by some that the physician plays a major role in determining the quantity of services to be provided [6, for example].

The concern over cost among consumers has been reinforced in recent years by that of third-party payers, particularly the government. Open-ended commitments to finance services have been followed by very large increases in price and expenditures; these increases have stimulated efforts to uncover their causes and to develop techniques for moderating them in the future.

This study, which is part of that effort, is composed of two principal parts. The first provides a statistical decomposition of the growth of per capita expenditures at the national level. Major attention is focused on the sharp differences in the rate of change of this variable between the subperiods 1948-56 (4.1 per cent per

---

[1] The comparable 1948-69 growth was 260 per cent for gross national product, 230 per cent for personal consumption expenditures, and 330 per cent for all services (except housing).

annum) and 1956-66 (6.6 per cent per annum). Possible reasons for this difference are explored through an examination of changes in price, insurance coverage, income, population, number and type of physicians, and medical technology. Problems of definition and measurement are discussed and some tentative inferences are drawn.

The second part is concerned with the development and testing of a formal model to analyze the behavior of physicians and patients. Cross-sectional (state) data for 1966 are used to gain an understanding of variations in quantity of services per capita, physicians per capita, quantity of services per physician, and insurance coverage. The consequences for health of differences in the quantity of physicians' services are also explored.

The principal limitations of the study are attributable to the paucity of available data. In our analyses we are frequently forced to exclude certain variables that seem appropriate on a priori grounds, or to include series that are only partially indicative of the variables actually desired. For instance, nearly all of the analysis is limited to physicians in private practice. Data on expenditures for services rendered by salaried members of hospital staffs are not available. Even for private physicians the breakdown of expenditures into price and quantity components is based on indirect estimates rather than precise direct measures. Finally, it should be noted that this paper is not intended to review systematically the literature on physicians' services, although we do consider the views of other observers in the formulation of hypotheses.[2]

Summary of Findings

The most striking finding of this study is that supply factors (technology and number of physicians) appear to be of decisive importance in determining the utilization of and expenditures for physicians' services. This conclusion stands in sharp contrast to the widely held belief that utilization and expenditures are determined by the patient, and that information about income, insurance coverage, and price is sufficient to explain and predict changes in demand.

The data we present in Part 1 show that the shift in the growth rate of physicians' services[3] per capita from −0.4 per cent per annum in 1948-56 to 3.0 per cent per annum in 1956-66 is more closely related to the changing nature of medical technology and to shifts in the number of physicians than to conventional demand variables. It seems to us that estimates of future "needs" for physicians are likely to be unreliable unless one can predict the nature and extent of future changes in medical science. That there will be such changes is certain; whether they will be of a type that economizes on the use of physicians' services (such as the antibiotic drugs) or whether they will increase the requirements for physicians (such as organ transplants) is of crucial importance. Furthermore, the "need" for physicians' services should not be treated as synonymous with the "need" for physicians; the record shows that the quantity of service per physician has been rising over time, and at a variable rate.

When we turn to an examination of variations in demand, holding technology constant (in the cross-sectional analysis of Part 2), we find additional support for the view that the number of physicians has a significant influence on utilization, quite apart from the effect of numbers on demand via lower fees. Indeed, we find that the elasticities of demand with respect to income, price, and insurance are all small relative to the direct effect of the number of physicians on demand. Of course, the emphasis we give to supply does not deny an independent role for demand entirely, especially when the patient is faced with major changes in the net price of care, such as those created by the introduction of Medicare and Medicaid.

Because physicians can and do determine the demand for their own services to a considerable extent, we should be wary of plans which assume that the cost of medical care would be reduced by increasing the supply of physicians. Our analysis suggests that such increases would at best have limited impact on price, though they would result in substantial increases in utilization. In estimating the social value of increased utilization,

---

[2] For comparisons of our formulations and conclusions with those of other investigators, see our bibliography [4], [7], [15], [16], [17], [28], [37], [41].

[3] "Quantity" is measured by deflating expenditures by an estimate of the average price actually received by physicians. It is not equivalent to number of visits because it also reflects shifts in the type of physician visited (specialist or G.P.) as well as in the quantity of tests, x-rays, and other services provided in the course of the average visit.

however, note should be taken of our finding (in section 2.6) that variations across states in the quantity of physicians' services appear to have little or no effect on either infant mortality or the overall death rate. Of course, an increase in physician supply has other effects that should be considered. The subjective utility derived from the consumption of physicians' services is likely to rise as physicians devote more time and personalized attention to each complaint, and the indirect costs incurred by patients will fall as general access to physicians improves. The subjective qualitative aspects of physicians' services are not considered in this paper.

Given the importance of supply, it is of interest to ask what factors determine it. The cross-sectional analysis throws some light on physicians' locational decisions. They seem to be attracted by higher prices for their services, by medical schools and hospital beds, and by the level of educational, cultural, and recreational opportunities indicated by the average income of the population. We did not find any evidence for the theory that encouraging more state residents to enter medical schools pays off in terms of more physicians returning to practice in their state of origin. Also, physicians do not show any special preference for states with low health levels. This absence of what some might regard as "professional responsibility" in choice of location stands in contrast to the behavior of physicians already established in a given location. We find that physicians practicing in states where the physician-population ratio is low *do* provide more services apart from any price considerations. Indeed, given location, there is no evidence to show that higher prices induce additional services from physicians; there is some reason to believe that they may have the opposite effect.

One finding in which we have considerable confidence deserves special mention because it reveals the unusual nature of the market for physicians' services. We refer to the fact that states with high quantity of service per capita (Q^*) have relatively low quantity of service per physician (Q/MD). The coefficient of correlation in 1966 was -0.5. The quantity series is admittedly imperfect, but errors of measurement in that variable would tend to produce a positive correlation between Q^* and Q/MD. There is good reason to believe, therefore, that the true correlation is even more negative than -0.5. Such a relationship is very surprising under either one of the following two interpretations of the Q/MD variable. If it is regarded as a measure of the average size of the "firm,"[4] we would expect a positive correlation with quantity per capita. If we regard it as a partial productivity measure, we would also expect a positive correlation with quantity per capita. These expectations are based on experience with many other industries [39, for example]. The negative relationship observed in this industry may be attributed to the behavior of physicians. Where these are relatively numerous they both increase the demand for their collective services and cut back on the amount of service each one individually provides. Where physicians are scarce the reverse occurs. The result is a strong negative correlation between Q^* and Q/MD.

Having set forth what we believe to be reasonable inferences from the data we have examined, we hasten to remind the reader of the caveats mentioned throughout the paper. The statistical experiments performed in Part 2 cannot be regarded as definitive; obvious weaknesses in the data and possible shortcomings in the specification of the model suggest that the empirical findings should be regarded as highly tentative. Given the data limitations, the chief contributions of Part 2 are the development of a comprehensive model of the market for physicians' services and the development of a technique for estimating quantity and price by state.

Additional research is clearly essential in order to predict accurately the consequences of proposed changes in the financing and organization of medical care, and the availability of relevant, reliable data will be of critical importance to the success of that research. Considering the magnitude of health care expenditures (over $70 billion per annum), strenuous efforts to make such data available would seem justified.

---

[4] This would be the case if all physicians had solo practices.

1

Differences Over Time, 1948-68:
A Statistical Decomposition

In Part 1 we examine the rate of change in expenditures and related variables over the period 1948-68 and for subperiods 1948-56, 1956-66, and 1966-68.[1] The growth rate for any period is calculated by treating the variable under study as a logarithmic function of time and fitting a least-squares regression through all the annual observations. The regression coefficient of time is equivalent to average percentage rate of change continuously compounded.

The rate of change in different subperiods varied greatly for expenditures per capita, quantity per capita, and quantity per physician. Most of Part 1 is devoted to explaining these differences. This involves an examination of changes in price, insurance coverage, income, demographic structure, number and type of physicians, and medical technology.

1.1 Expenditures

Problems of Definition

It is difficult to specify what should be included among expenditures for "physicians' services." The principal reason is the central role that physicians play in the entire field of health services. When a patient places himself in the care of a physician, he frequently is purchasing a wide range of diagnostic and therapeutic services, some of which will be rendered personally by the physician but many of which will involve the use of capital equipment or auxiliary personnel functioning under the control of the physician. For example, a physician may order several tests and x-rays as part of a physical examination. Are the costs of these tests and x-rays to be considered part of the cost of the physician's service? Most students of medical care would say they should be because the tests and x-rays are an integral part of the examination. However, the official statistics of the Department of Health, Education, and Welfare treat such costs in this fashion only if payment is part of the gross receipts of the physician. The very same tests and x-rays that are included if the patient

visits the doctor's office may not be included if the doctor treats the patient in the hospital. Furthermore, though the operating room is an integral part of the service rendered by a surgeon, expenditures for its use (and for associated nursing personnel) are not considered part of the cost of the surgeon's services.

Not only is the classification of auxiliary services ambiguous, but the measurement of direct personal service rendered by physicians is also clouded by institutional arrangements. The Department of Health, Education, and Welfare expenditures statistics essentially cover only physicians in private practice; the cost of services rendered by physicians who are salaried members of hospital staffs is not included. During the period under study the percentage of active physicians who were salaried members of hospital staffs rose from 12 to 21.

In this study we are concerned with expenditures for services rendered by physicians in private practice. Series dealing with price, visits, number of physicians, et cetera are chosen to conform as closely as possible to this universe of expenditures. Physicians' services thus defined have accounted for between one-fifth and one-fourth of all health expenditures since 1948, with no trend discernible in the size of the share. They accounted for one per cent of the gross national product in 1948 and 1.4 per cent in 1969. Thus, there has been a 40 per cent increase in the share of the nation's resources devoted to this service in only two decades.

The exclusion of salaried hospital physicians results in an underestimate of the rate of growth of expenditures for all physicians' services. We have made several alternative estimates of the growth in expenditures for salaried hospital physicians; they suggest that the underestimate is on the order of 0.2 to 0.4 per cent per annum for 1948-68. Inasmuch as the growth in relative importance of hospital-based physicians was fairly uniform over the two decades, however, their omission is inconsequential for the analysis of differences between subperiods.

Problems of Measurement

The Department of Health, Education, and Welfare series on expenditures for physicians' services exhibits

---

[1] The initial and terminal years for the subperiods—1948, 1956, 1966, and 1968—were all years of high levels of economic activity (as indicated by the unemployment rates in those years, which were 3.8, 4.1, 3.8, and 3.6 per cent, respectively).

striking year-to-year fluctuations, as shown in Chart 1. These erratic changes reflect similar movements in the gross receipts figures reported for physicians in private practice by the Internal Revenue Service, which form the basis for the HEW estimates.

Chart 1

Percentage Changes in Expenditures per Capita for Physicians' Services, 1948-68

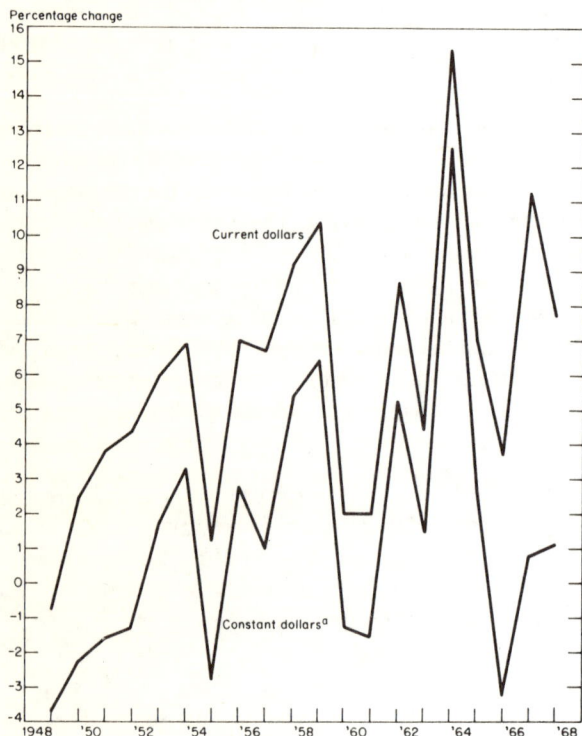

Source: See Appendix A.

aDeflated by average price received (i.e., customary price adjusted for estimated effects of changes in insurance coverage; see p. 7).

Part of the erratic movement in the expenditures data appears to be related to inexplicable variations in the number of physicians filing income tax returns. For instance, between 1963 and 1964 the number of physicians filing increased by 8.0 per cent. The following year the number decreased by 2.1 per cent. The American Medical Association's series on M.D.s in private practice, believed to be reasonably accurate, does not show any annual swings of this nature. Over periods as long as five to ten years, the IRS and AMA series on number of physicians show almost exactly the same rates of change.

It seems likely that there are substantial errors in some of the year-to-year movements [28], and this

raises grave doubts about the value of econometric analyses based on annual changes. Because the average rate of change over several years is probably much less subject to error, we shall give major attention to such changes in this study.

The Data

Table 1 presents annual data on expenditures for private physicians in both total and per capita form. Table 2 shows the average annual rates of change, which are our primary interest. We see that there was a sharp acceleration in the rate of growth between the major subperiods 1948-56 and 1956-66, and a further acceleration in 1966-68. This conclusion is not sensitive to the choice of initial and terminal years; the same pattern of acceleration is evident if we use 1955 or 1957 instead of 1956, or if we use 1965 or 1967 instead of 1966. The figures in parentheses under the growth rates are their standard errors.[2] By applying a variant of the t test, we find that the differences between the subperiods are statistically significant even though there are relatively

TABLE 1

Expenditures for Physicians' Services, 1948-68

Year	Total (Millions of $)	Per Capita ($)
1948	2,611	17.99
1949	2,633	17.84
1950	2,747	18.29
1951	2,868	18.99
1952	3,042	19.83
1953	3,278	21.02
1954	3,574	22.47
1955	3,689	22.73
1956	4,067	24.31
1957	4,419	25.94
1958	4,909	28.32
1959	5,481	31.27
1960	5,684	31.90 ·
1961	5,895	32.53
1962	6,498	35.35
1963	6,891	36.92
1964	8,065	42.59
1965	8,745	45.57
1966	9,156	47.25
1967	10,287	52.57
1968	11,188	56.63

Source: See Appendix A.

[2] The growth rate is the regression coefficient b in the equation

$$\ln Y = a + bT$$

where T equals time.

TABLE 2

Rates of Change of Expenditures for Physicians' Services, 1948-68

(per cent per annum continuously compounded)

	1948-56	1956-66	1966-68	1948-68
Total	5.7 (0.4)	8.1 (0.3)	10.0 (0.9)	7.6 (0.2)
Per capita	4.1 (0.3)	6.6 (0.3)	9.1 (0.9)	6.0 (0.2)

Note: Standard errors of rates of change are shown in parentheses.

Source: Table 1.

few observations.[3] Comparing the 1948-56 growth in per capita expenditures with that of 1956-66, the probability of obtaining a difference as large as the one observed as a result of chance is less than 0.01. For the comparison of 1956-66 with 1966-68, $p = 0.05$.

In the analysis that follows we shall concentrate on explaining these significant disparities in rates of growth, especially those between 1948-56 and 1956-66.[4] Heavy reliance on 1966-68 does not seem warranted, given the brevity of the period, the paucity of data, and the likelihood that some of the available data will be revised. Nevertheless, section 1.11 offers a brief discussion of this period. Here our first task is to separate expenditures into its price and quantity components.

1.2 Price and Insurance

The discussions of price and insurance fall logically together; there are several concepts of price that are relevant to our analysis, and the differences in their trends are closely tied to trends in insurance for physicians' services.

---

[3]The standard error of the difference between two coefficients is equal to the difference divided by the square root of the sum of the squared standard errors of each coefficient. Thus

$$t = \frac{b_1 - b_2}{\sqrt{S_{b_1} + S_{b_2}}}.$$

[4]Medicare and Medicaid were introduced in 1966; thus it is a logical break point in the time series.

Customary Price

The Bureau of Labor Statistics collects information every month from physicians concerning their "usual and customary fee," and this information forms the basis for the physicians' fee component that goes into the medical care portion of the Consumer Price Index. The customary fee index is a weighted average of standard fees charged for an office visit by "family physicians" (formerly "general practitioners"), for an appendectomy, and for other specified categories of visits. This index may behave very differently from an index that measures the average price actually received by physicians, or from one that measures the net price paid by patients.

Average Price Received

The average price received may deviate from the customary or nominal price for two principal reasons. First, physicians do not charge all their patients the customary fee [26]; they may charge poor patients significantly lower fees and may treat some without any charge. Secondly, physicians do not collect 100 per cent of the fees they do charge.

One of the uses of the price index is to obtain a series of the real quantity of services by deflating the expenditures series. For such purposes the appropriate price series is one that measures the average price received by physicians, not the customary price. To the extent that physicians charge less than their customary fee and to the extent that they fail to collect all the fees they do charge, deflation of expenditures by the customary fee would result in a biased estimate of quantity.

Our approach to both these problems is based upon the assumption that a physician is more likely to charge his customary fee and more likely to collect his charges when the service is covered by insurance.[5] The extent of insurance coverage has two dimensions: the number of people carrying protection, and the average level of protection per person insured. In both aspects of

---

[5]This approach was proposed and applied by Martin S. Feldstein [16]. We have utilized additional data and relaxed some of his assumptions in deriving our average price series. An alternative approach employed by Klarman et al. [28] utilizes direct estimates of changes in collection ratios, but makes no adjustment for deviations between customary and actual charges.

coverage dramatic increases were recorded during the postwar period. The number of persons with private insurance coverage for physician expenses grew from approximately 34 million in 1948 to 160 million in 1968, and average annual benefits per insured rose from $4.61 to $23.57. The contrast between the initial and terminal years becomes even greater when the Medicare and Medicaid populations are included among the insured and expenditures made under these programs are added to those covered by private insurance. All third-party payments together accounted for 11 per cent of expenditures in 1948 and 57 per cent twenty years later (Chart 2).

Chart 2
Growth of Third-Party Payment for
Physicians' Services, 1948-68

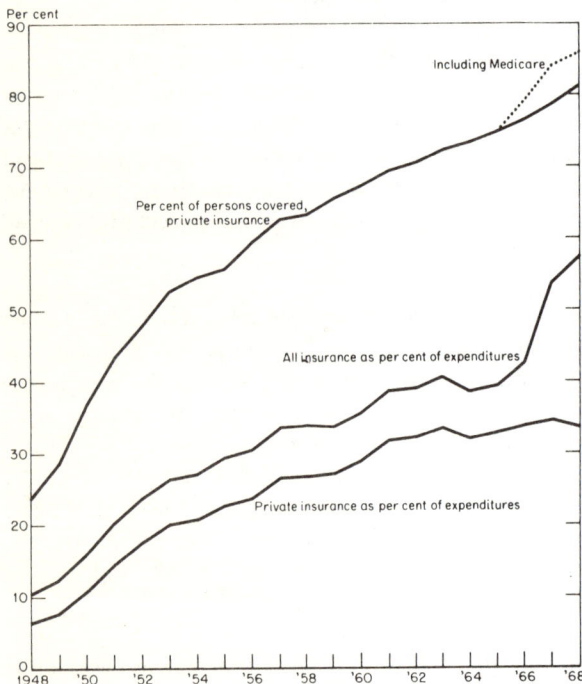

Source: See Appendix A.

The ratio of average price to customary price in any year depends upon the proportions of insured and uninsured in the population (I and N), the utilization per insured relative to utilization per uninsured (U), the fraction of customary price paid by insured persons (K), and the fraction of customary price paid by uninsured persons (k). More exactly,

$$\frac{AP}{CP} = \frac{U \cdot I \cdot K + N \cdot k}{U \cdot I + N}.$$

If everyone were fully insured $(N=0, K=1)$, average price would equal customary price. Average price approaches customary price with increases in the percentage insured of the population, in the utilization ratio, and in the average payment ratio of insured persons. It is assumed that K varies with the fraction of insured persons' utilization covered by insurance. Starting from a lower limit of k, it reaches an upper limit of 1.0 when all services purchased by insured persons are fully covered. k is assumed to remain constant over time at 0.67. (The basis for our estimates of U, K, and k and the sources of data employed in the application of this formula are given in Appendix B.)

According to our formula, the ratio of average price to customary price rose from 0.72 in 1948 to 0.89 in 1968. The average annual rate of change of average price from 1948-68 was 4.2 per cent, compared with 3.2 per cent for customary price. The disparity in the growth rates of the two price series was larger before 1956 than after that date. This conforms with the results of Klarman et al., based on estimates of physician collection ratios [28], and of Martin Feldstein [16].

Net Price

While the growth of insurance coverage tends to raise the average price received by physicians relative to the customary price charged, it has the opposite effect on the net price paid by patients. To the patient, an increase in the share of the bill covered by insurance appears as a decrease in the price he pays. Following Martin Feldstein, we calculate net price as equal to average price multiplied by the fraction of expenditures the patient must pay directly:

$$NP = AP \cdot \left(\frac{\text{expenditures} - \text{third-party payments}}{\text{expenditures}} \right).$$

The three price series for physicians' services are presented in Tables 3 and 4 along with the Consumer Price Index for all goods and services. Table 4 shows that net price rose at the rate of 1.3 per cent per annum from 1948 to 1968. Its fastest growth was during 1956-66, and after 1966 it actually declined as a result of the large increase in third-party payments by government.

When net price rises more slowly than the price of other goods and services, physicians' services are relatively cheaper, and we might expect an increase in the quantity demanded. When net price rises faster than the

TABLE 3

Price Indexes of Physicians' Services and All Goods and Services, 1948-68

(1956=100)

Year	Physicians' Services			All Goods and Services
	Customary Price	Average Price Received	Net Price Paid	Consumer Price Index
1948 ..	79.3	71.0	91.1	88.5
1949 ..	80.7	73.1	92.1	87.6
1950 ..	82.5	76.6	92.4	88.5
1951 ..	85.1	80.8	92.6	95.6
1952 ..	88.8	85.6	93.6	97.7
1953 ..	91.2	89.2	94.2	98.4
1954 ..	93.8	92.3	96.5	98.8
1955 ..	97.1	96.1	97.1	98.5
1956 ..	100.0	100.0	100.0	100.0
1957 ..	104.3	105.7	100.4	103.5
1958 ..	107.9	109.4	103.7	106.3
1959 ..	111.5	113.6	108.1	107.2
1960 ..	114.3	117.4	108.9	108.9
1961 ..	117.2	121.6	106.8	110.0
1962 ..	120.7	125.5	109.9	111.3
1963 ..	123.4	129.1	110.2	112.7
1964 ..	126.5	132.2	117.0	114.1
1965 ..	131.1	137.8	120.1	116.0
1966 ..	138.6	147.6	122.2	119.4
1967 ..	148.4	163.0	108.1	122.8
1968 ..	156.7	173.7	106.6	128.0

Source: See Appendixes A and B.

TABLE 4

Rates of Change of Prices of Physicians' Services and All Goods and Services, 1948-68

(per cent per annum continuously compounded)

	1948-56	1956-66	1966-68	1948-68
Customary price	3.0 (0.1)	3.0 (0.1)	6.1 (0.4)	3.2 (0.1)
Average price received.	4.4 (0.1)	3.6 (0.1)	8.1 (1.0)	4.2 (0.1)
Net price paid	1.1 (0.1)	1.9 (0.2)	-6.8 (3.0)	1.3 (0.1)
Consumer Price Index.	1.8 (0.3)	1.5 (0.1)	3.5 (0.4)	1.7 (0.1)

Note: Standard errors of rates of change are shown in parentheses.

Source: Table 3.

considered as an exogenous phenomenon rather than as a direct result of an increased demand for medical care. Given the additional coverage, patients found that the net price to them of medical care was lower, and they responded by demanding more care. This increase in demand resulted in higher expenditures.

With respect to the period 1966-68, we find that this hypothesis fits well with the observed data. The rapid growth in expenditures coincided with a major increase in third-party payments, and, indeed, there appears to have been an absolute as well as a relative decrease in direct spending by patients after 1966 (see Tables 5 and 6).

On the other hand, this hypothesis is of no help in explaining the difference in growth rates before and after 1956. In fact, the relative growth of insurance was far more important in the first than in the second subperiod. We see that the differential between 1956-66 and 1948-56 in growth of direct expenditures by patients was greater (4.3 per cent per annum) than the differential for all expenditures (2.5 per cent per annum). Thus, this approach yields the same conclusion as the comparison of net price with the Consumer Price Index, namely, that differential changes in insurance cannot explain the upsurge of utilization after 1956.

Consumer Price Index, we might expect the reverse. The magnitude of the effect is determined by: (1) the differential change in price and (2) the elasticity of demand for physicians' services with respect to changes in price. Most observers believe this elasticity to be quite small. If so, differential price changes will not have much effect on demand. The main point to be noted, however, is that whatever the size of the effect, Table 4 shows that it would be in the direction of *lowering* demand in 1956-66 relative to 1948-56 or 1966-68.

Impact of Insurance on Growth of Expenditures

One of the factors commonly believed to be responsible for the sharp growth of expenditures for physicians' services is insurance (both private and public). According to this view, the growth of insurance coverage should be

TABLE 5

Relative Importance of Insurance for Physicians' Services, 1948-68

Year	Per Cent of Population with Private Insurance	Per Cent of Expenditures Paid by		
		Private Insurance	Public Programs	Patients Directly
1948	23.6	6.1	4.4	89.5
1949	28.1	7.4	4.8	87.8
1950	36.4	10.7	5.2	84.1
1951	43.3	14.4	5.7	79.9
1952	47.7	17.7	6.0	76.3
1953	52.5	20.0	6.3	73.7
1954	54.6	20.6	6.4	73.0
1955	55.5	22.8	6.7	70.5
1956	59.5	23.5	6.7	69.8
1957	62.7	26.7	7.0	66.3
1958	63.1	26.8	7.1	66.1
1959	65.6	26.9	6.8	66.3
1960	67.1	28.9	6.4	64.7
1961	69.3	31.9	6.9	61.2
1962	70.5	32.1	6.9	61.0
1963	72.2	33.5	6.9	59.6
1964	73.1	32.0	6.3	61.7
1965	74.9	32.9	6.3	60.8
1966	76.5	33.7	8.6	57.7
1967	78.8	34.4	19.3	46.3
1968	80.8	33.6	23.6	42.8

Note: Per cent of population covered by Medicare and/or private insurance in 1966-68: 1966, 79.1; 1967, 84.0; 1968, 85.9.

Source: See Appendix A.

TABLE 6

Rates of Change of Third-Party and Direct Expenditures for Physicians' Services, 1948-68

(per cent per annum continuously compounded)

Per Capita Expenditures	1948-56	1956-66	1966-68	1948-68
Third parties	17.7 (1.4)	9.4 (0.2)	24.2 (6.0)	12.5 (0.5)
Patients directly . . .	0.7 (0.5)	5.0 (0.5)	-5.9 (3.2)	3.2 (0.3)

Note: Standard errors of rates of change are shown in parentheses.

Source: See Appendix A.

1.3 Quantity of Physicians' Services

Deflation of expenditures by average price yields a "quantity" series. This is not necessarily equivalent to a measure of the number of physician visits, since it includes an implicit adjustment for shifts in the type of physician visit and in the amount of auxiliary services (e.g., tests and x-rays) performed at each visit.[6] In effect, the various types of service and types of visits are weighted by their respective price ratios.[7]

This measure of quantity does not take into account any changes over time in the "quality" associated with a given service from a given type of physician. For instance, a routine office visit to a general practitioner would count as the same quantity in 1968 as in 1948 even though the "output," in the sense of improved health, might be different as the result of advances in medical knowledge, new drugs, et cetera. Similarly, the series does not take into account any changes in amenities, physician behavior, or other aspects of service that could affect the utility derived by the patient from the visit.

Table 7 shows that quantity per capita grew at an average annual rate of only 1.8 per cent between 1948 and 1968. Most of the growth of expenditures during that period (7.6 per cent per annum) is accounted for by changes in customary price (3.2 per cent per annum), the ratio of average price to customary price (1.0 per cent per annum), and the size of the population (1.6 per cent per annum).

Comparison of the subperiods reveals some interesting differences. During 1948-56, quantity per capita actually declined at the rate of 0.4 per cent per annum. This decline is not significantly different from a zero rate of change according to conventional statistical tests, but is very significantly different from the 3.0 per cent rate of advance registered during 1956-66. The practical significance of the shift in growth rates is enormous. If quantity per capita had continued to change at its 1948-56 rate after 1956, the average physician would

---

[6] An analysis of changes in quantity per physician and per visit is presented in section 1.9.

[7] Use of these implicit price weights might be questioned because of imperfections in the market for physicians' services, but there are no alternative data that would permit a more direct approach to weighting different services. Moreover, the errors introduced by imperfect weights are likely to be very small relative to the errors in the original expenditures series.

TABLE 7

Rates of Change of Quantity of Physicians' Services, Personal
Income, and Predicted Expenditures and Visits, 1948-68

(per cent per annum continuously compounded)

	1948-56	1956-66	1966-68	1948-68
Quantity of services total.	1.3 (0.4)	4.5 (0.3)	1.9 (0.1)	3.4 (0.2)
per capita.	-0.4 (0.4)	3.0 (0.3)	0.9 (0.1)	1.8 (0.2)
Real disposable personal income per capita	2.2 (0.2)	2.4 (0.3)	2.6 (0.1)	2.2[a] (0.1)
Predicted expenditures per capita based on changes in age-sex structure of population	-0.2	-0.1	0.2	-0.1
Predicted visits per capita based on changes in age-sex structure of population	0.0	-0.1	0.0	0.0

Note: Standard errors of rates of change are shown in parentheses.

Source: See Appendix A and Table 8.

[a]The apparent inconsistency between the rate of change for the entire period and the subperiods is due to the fact that this series shows a slight decline from the final years of the first period to the initial years of the second period. Therefore, a line fitted through the period as a whole shows a growth rate no greater than that of the slower of the two subperiods.

have 40 per cent less business today than he actually has. After 1966 the growth rate of quantity per capita fell sharply once more, though we must point out that possible errors in either the expenditures or price series, or both, could introduce substantial errors into the growth rate for a period as short as three years.

In our judgment, the large difference in the growth rate of quantity per capita observed between 1948-56 and 1956-66 cannot be attributed to errors of measurement but represents a true shift in actual utilization of physicians' services. The necessity to explain this shift poses a major problem for health economists, one that has not been adequately resolved by earlier studies. The preceding section demonstrates that the shift cannot be attributed to changes in price or insurance. Next we shall

investigate whether it can be attributed to changes in income or in the demographic structure of the population.

1.4   Income

Other things being equal, the faster the growth of income, the more rapidly the demand for physicians' services should rise. Table 7 shows that real disposable income per capita did grow more rapidly in 1956-66 than in 1948-56, but the difference is only 0.2 per cent per annum, and not statistically significant. If we assume that the income elasticity[8] for physicians' services is as high as 1.0 (most observers believe it to be less than that [4, 17]), we could attribute 0.2 of a percentage point of the differential change in quantity per capita to changes in the growth of income.

It should be noted that over the entire twenty-year period, real disposable personal income per capita grew more rapidly than did quantity per capita (2.2 per cent versus 1.8 per cent). However, to the extent that growth in expenditures is underestimated through the omission of salaried hospital physicians, so is growth in quantity per capita. It is probable that the quantity of all physicians' services grew at very nearly the same rate as real disposable income.

It has been suggested that, in addition to changes in the average level of income, shifts in the distribution of income could also affect the demand for physicians' services. During the period under study, however, the degree of inequality in personal income was remarkably stable. (See [9], [38].)

1.5   Demographic Structure

It is well known that utilization of physicians' services varies with age and sex. Generally speaking, utilization is high in infancy, low during childhood and adolescence, low for males of working age, high for females of childbearing age, and relatively high for both sexes in old age.

In order to determine whether shifts in the demographic structure of the population could account for

---

[8] The income elasticity of demand is defined as the percentage change in quantity associated with a one per cent change in income.

part of the shift in per capita utilization, either overall or for subperiods, we made two sets of calculations. The percentage of the total population in each of twelve age-sex classes was computed for 1948, 1956, 1966, and 1968. The distributions for each year were then weighted, first by (a) average per capita expenditures for each age-sex class in 1962, and then by (b) average number of per capita visits for each age-sex class in 1963-64.

The results, presented in Tables 7 and 8, indicate that shifts in the age-sex structure of the population probably had a negligible effect on the utilization of physicians' services over the two decades. When the population distribution is weighted by expenditures, the data lead us to expect a 0.1 per cent per annum decline in 1948-56 relative to 1956-66, and when the weighting is done by visits, the reverse is true. We should note, however, a predicted 0.3 per cent per annum faster increase for the 1966-68 period than for 1956-66 when expenditures are used for weights.

1.6   Recapitulation: Comparison of 1956-66 with 1948-56

Table 9 provides a brief recapitulation of our attempt to explain differential trends in the first two subperiods. The differential in expenditures growth per capita of 2.5 per cent per annum can be decomposed into a differential in average price (−0.8) and in quantity per capita (3.4).

To explain the differential change in quantity per capita we first consider the movement of net price paid by patients relative to the Consumer Price Index for all goods and services. As explained in section 1.2, this movement was of a kind to decrease demand in 1956-66 relative to 1948-56. In order to arrive at a *minimum* estimate of the unexplained residual, and because of uncertainty regarding the price elasticity of demand, no quantitative estimate is made of this effect. We simply note that it would be in a negative direction.

TABLE 8

Predicted Effects of Changes in Age-Sex Structure of Population on Utilization of Physicians' Services,

1948-68

Age-Sex Groups	Expenditures[a] (1962 $ per Capita)	Visits (Number per Capita, 1963-64)	1948	1956	1966	1968
Males			*Per Cent of Population*			
<5	$28	5.7	10.6	11.4	10.6	9.7
5-14	21	2.9	16.7	19.4	21.3	21.4
15-24	24	3.2	15.6	13.4	16.2	16.8
25-44	37	3.4	29.2	27.7	23.7	23.7
45-64	58	4.4	20.7	20.0	19.9	20.0
≥65	62	6.1	7.2	8.0	8.3	8.4
Females						
<5	25	5.3	10.0	10.8	9.7	8.9
5-14	19	2.7	15.9	18.4	19.8	19.8
15-24	59	5.2	15.5	12.9	15.8	16.4
25-44	64	5.6	30.3	28.2	23.7	23.6
45-64	64	5.5	20.5	20.5	20.5	20.7
≥65	61	7.2	7.8	9.2	10.5	10.7
			Predicted Levels			
Expenditures[b]			$44.77	$43.99	$43.63	$43.84
Visits[c]			4.54	4.54	4.51	4.51

Sources: See Appendix A.

[a]Weights based on age groups <6, 6-16, 17-24, 25-44, 45-64, and ≥65 years.
[b]Standardized according to 1962 levels and patterns of expenditures.
[c]Standardized according to 1963-64 levels and patterns of visits.

TABLE 9

Comparison of 1956-66 With 1948-56, Expenditures
per Capita and Related Variables

(per cent per annum continuously compounded)

	1948-56	1956-66	1956-66 minus 1948-56
Expenditures per capita...	4.1	6.6	2.5[a]
Average price.......	4.4	3.6	-0.8
Customary price ...	3.0	3.0	0.0
Ratio of AP to CP ..	1.4	0.6	-0.8
Quantity per capita ...	-0.4	3.0	3.4[a]
Explanatory variables			*Effects*
Net price relative to price of all goods and services			Negative
Real per capita disposable income			0.2
Distribution of income .			Negligible
Age-sex structure			0.1
Minimum unexplained residual			3.1

Sources: Tables 2 and 4.

[a]This differs slightly from the sum of its two components because of rounding.

The disposable income effect is based on an observed differential of 0.2 per cent per annum in the growth of per capita real disposable income and an assumption of unitary (1.0) income elasticity of demand. This probably also errs on the conservative side; if, as most observers believe, the income elasticity is below 1.0, the effect would be less than 0.2.

The bases for our estimates of very small effects resulting from changes in distribution of income and age-sex structure are explained in 1.4 and 1.5. Thus, we are left with a minimum unexplained residual of 3.1 per cent, which, we must emphasize, is highly significant in all senses of the term.

1.7   Technological Change

Conventional demand variables do not explain the sharp increase in the growth rate of utilization in 1956-66 over the previous period. We believe that some insight into this phenomenon can be gained by an examination of changes in medical technology and of the consequences of these changes for health.

Michael Grossman has shown that the demand for medical care (or any component thereof) can fruitfully be treated as being *derived* from the demand for *health* [22]. Most people do not consume physicians' services as an end in itself but rather for their presumed value in curing disease, relieving pain, et cetera. The degree to which physicians can meet that underlying demand for health is likely to depend upon the state of medical technology. Some advances in medical science might require very little physician input to implement; others might require a great deal. A detailed look at changes in medical technology is beyond the scope of this paper, but a brief review of major innovations is appropriate.

The late 1940's and early 1950's were marked by the introduction and widespread diffusion of many new drugs that were extremely effective against influenza, pneumonia, tuberculosis, and other infectious diseases which had previously played a large role in mortality and morbidity. The advances in drug therapy are well known and need be mentioned only briefly here. Penicillin was discovered in 1928, but mass production and distribution came much later. For instance, between 1945 and 1950 the annual production of penicillin increased from 12,000 to 330,000 pounds [13]. Streptomycin was discovered in 1943 and widespread distribution came several years later. The year 1948 marked the introduction of the first broad spectrum antibiotic, chlortetracycline, and this was soon followed by chloramphenicol. In 1950 oxytetracycline was introduced, and another major broad spectrum antibiotic, tetracycline, appeared in 1953. These antibiotics had a pronounced impact on the length and severity of infectious diseases. The use of para-aminosalicylic acid (late 1940's) and isoniazid (1952) in the treatment of tuberculosis also had considerable effect.

Since 1956, there has not been a similar improvement in the ability of physicians to alter health. Those advances that have occurred, such as renal dialysis, cancer chemotherapy, and open heart surgery, have typically been of a kind that make for only marginal improvements in general health indexes, despite occasionally dramatic effects in particular cases.

The differential health impact of medical advances in the two periods is implicit in the behavior of death rates

(Table 10 and Chart 3). Mortality declined for several years after 1948, but the decline ended in the middle 1950's. Since then, crude death rates and many of the age-specific rates have tended to remain rather stable. The early declines were particularly dramatic for infectious diseases. They were also relatively greatest for the younger age groups.

In our view the improvement in health prior to 1956 which resulted from application of the new medical technology helps to explain the decline in per capita utilization of physicians' services in those years. The absence of comparable health effects accruing from the medical advances of later years suggests that the demand for physicians' services might have leveled off; the health factor alone, however, cannot account for the marked rise in demand from 1956 to 1966. To understand that, we must also take into consideration the nature of the technological changes. In general, the early advances tended to be physician-saving, while those of the latter period were characteristically physician-using. Physician time was, of course, required for the prescription and administration of the "wonder drugs," but they frequently produced rapid improvement in health, thereby reducing total utilization of physicians' services. Since

Chart 3

Indexes of Health, 1948-68

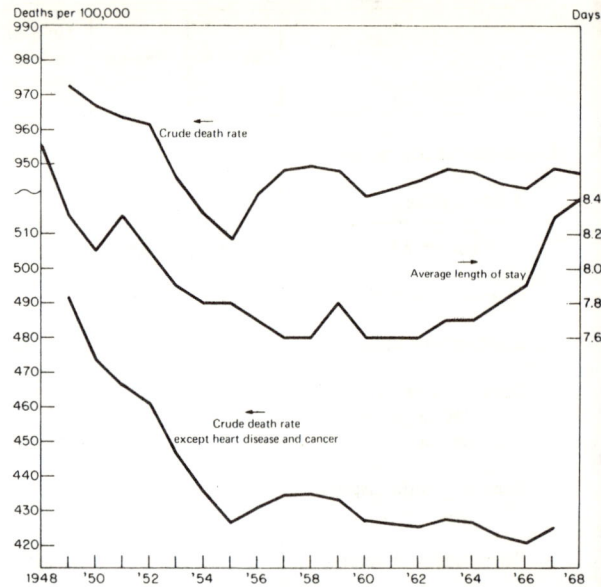

Note: Data smoothed by three-term moving average.
Source: See Appendix A.

1956, most medical advances have required substantial inputs of physician time for their implementation and have not had such pronounced effects on health. The result has been a rapid growth in utilization.

Evidence supporting our hypothesis can be found in the behavior of the average length of stay in short-term general hospitals. This statistic declined from 8.7 days in 1948 to 7.7 days in 1956. After 1956, average stay leveled off and then started to rise, reaching 7.9 days in 1966.[9] Also, hospital days per capita (admissions times average length of stay) were relatively stable in the first period, but rose appreciably in the second. The population's health did not worsen after 1956, but more cases became treatable and the average time of treatment rose. The increase in hospitalization was associated with increased utilization of physicians' services because the new technology required large inputs of both.

Thus, we postulate a latent demand for health, which appropriate technological change can transform into a market demand for services producing health. It was impossible to purchase a measles vaccination or heart-

TABLE 10

Rates of Change of Death Rates and Hospital Use, 1948-68

(per cent per annum continuously compounded)

	1948-56[a]	1956-66	1966-68	1948-68[a]
Death rate, all causes .	-0.7 (0.2)	0.0 (0.1)	n. a.	-0.1 (0.1)
Death rate, all causes except heart disease and cancer	-2.0 (0.3)	-0.2 (0.2)	n. a.	-0.6 (0.1)
Average length of hospital stay	-1.3 (0.2)	0.2 (0.1)	3.1 (1.1)	-0.2 (0.1)
Hospital days per capita[b]	0.4 (0.2)	1.7 (0.1)	2.8 (0.9)	1.3 (0.1)

Note: Standard errors of rates of change are shown in parentheses.

Source: See Appendix A.

[a] Periods shown for death rates are 1949-56 and 1949-67.
[b] Nonfederal short-term general hospitals.

---

[9] The figure reached 8.3 in 1969, but this later increase was probably attributable to Medicare.

lung machine a quarter of a century ago for any price, but as soon as these products were technically available, a market demand for them rapidly materialized. In both periods under review, technological change expanded the range of services physicians offered, and this in itself should have led to a growth in demand for these services. One would expect this growth to be much greater in the second period than in the first because the early advances necessitated only small inputs of physician time to be implemented, while the later ones were highly physician-intensive. The improvement in health that resulted from the early advances was so great that it turned the anticipated slight rise in demand into a slight decline, since healthier people have less objective *need* for the services of physicians. The advances in the second period exerted no significant downward pressure on demand via better health, and the large rise did, in fact, materialize.

One modest test of the technology hypothesis is to look at what was happening to dentists' services during the same period. The factors affecting demand and supply in this market are, in many respects, similar to those affecting physicians' services, the most notable difference being that changes in the two technologies are relatively independent. If dental services showed patterns of change similar to physicians' services, we would be inclined to reject an explanation that gives major importance to advances in medical science. On the other hand, if dental services showed a markedly different pattern of change over time, the emphasis on technological change in medicine would receive some support.

The data presented in Table 11 strongly confirm the latter position. Expenditures, customary fees, quantity

per capita, and quantity per dentist all rose more rapidly between 1948 and 1956 than during 1956-66.[10] This is in sharp contrast to physicians' services, where all these variables rose faster after 1956.

The deceleration in utilization of dental services may conceivably have been the result of the spread of fluoridation.[11] But even if this is the explanation, it only serves to strengthen the general point—the importance of technological change as a factor explaining secular changes in demand for health services.

1.8   The Supply of Physicians

No discussion of utilization of physicians' services can be complete without consideration of changes in the supply of physicians. There is no satisfactory annual series available covering physicians, but the AMA has published figures for certain benchmark years which we can use to calculate rates of change for the period 1949-67 and to estimate rates of change for the two major subperiods we are concerned with.[12]

According to Table 12, the number of active physicians per capita in the United States increased by almost 14 per cent from 1949 to 1967. The rate of increase, however, was very uneven by type of physician and type of practice. Particularly noteworthy was the decline in the percentage of physicians in private practice from 78.5 per cent in 1949 to 65.5 per cent in 1967. This was partly the result of a sharp increase in the relative importance of teaching, research, and other nonpatient-care activities. More important in absolute terms was the growth of salaried physicians in hospitals, including interns, residents, fellows, and regular full-time staff members. The rapid growth of specialists and the absolute decline in the number of general practitioners per capita should also be noted.

TABLE 11

Rates of Change of Dentists' Services, 1948-68

(per cent per annum continuously compounded)

	1948-56	1956-66	1966-68
Expenditures	8.3	6.1	9.9
Price (fee index)	3.2	2.4	5.1
Quantity (deflated expenditures)	5.1	3.7	4.8
Quantity per capita	3.5	2.1	3.7
Quantity per dentist	4.1	2.7	n. a.

Source: See Appendix A.

---

[10] The rapid increase in quantity per dentist in the first period might be attributable to the introduction of high speed drills.

[11] In 1948 fewer than half a million people were served by fluoridated water systems. By 1956 the figure had risen to 33 million, and by 1966, to 62 million. If several years of exposure to fluoridated water are required before the full impact on dental health is manifest, it is possible that fluoridation had a larger impact in the later than in the earlier period. See [51].

[12] 1949-57 is used as an approximation for 1948-56 and 1957-67 is used as an approximation for 1956-66.

TABLE 12

U.S. Physicians, by Type, Selected Years, 1949-67

	Number of Physicians per 100,000				Per Cent of Total Active Physicians			
	1949	1957	1963	1967	1949	1957	1963	1967
Total active physicians .	129.8	126.8	137.8	147.4	100.0	100.0	100.0	100.0
Federal	8.5	9.8	10.2	12.3	6.5	7.7	7.4	8.3
Nonfederal	121.3	117.0	127.6	135.1	93.4	92.3	92.6	91.7
Other than patient care	2.5	4.2	6.8	8.7	1.9	3.3	4.9	5.9
Patient care	118.8	112.8	120.8	126.4	91.5	89.0	87.7	85.8
Hospital service	16.9	21.3	25.3	29.9	13.0	16.8	18.4	20.3
Private practice	101.9	91.5	95.5	96.5	78.5	72.2	69.3	65.5
General practitioners .	64.7	47.8	36.5	31.8	49.8	37.7	26.5	21.6
Full-time specialists . . .	37.2	43.7	59.0	64.7	28.7	34.5	42.8	43.9

Source: See Appendix A.

When we consider changes in the number of private practice physicians per capita in the subperiods, we find a large difference between 1949-57 and 1957-67 (Table 13). The first subperiod shows a rate of change of −1.3 per cent per annum; the second shows an average annual increase of 0.5 per cent. The differential is even greater if we take account of the shift to specialists by treating them as the equivalent of 1.2 general practitioners. This weight is equal to the ratio of annual receipts of the average specialist relative to those of the average G.P. After this adjustment, we find that the differential in the rate of change between the two subperiods was on the order of 2.0 per cent per annum.

This change differential in the supply of physicians probably accounts for a portion of the unexplained differential in the growth of quantity per capita.[13] It must be stressed that the differential in supply can properly be treated as exogenous in this context (i.e., it is not the result of contemporaneous changes in demand). The number of physicians in practice in any year is largely determined by decisions made more than a decade previously.

What is the mechanism by which additional supply generates additional utilization? In "normal" economic

---

[13] See Part 2 for a test of this hypothesis.

TABLE 13

Average Annual Rates of Change of Private Practice Physicians, 1949-67

(per cent per annum continuously compounded)

	1949-57	1957-67	1949-67
Private practice physicians per capita	-1.3	0.5	-0.3
Weighted private practice physicians per capita (Specialists = 1.2 G.P.'s). . .	-1.1	0.9	0.0

Note: Rates of change from initial to terminal year.

Source: See Appendix A.

markets this occurs via price. The increase in supply depresses price and the lower price induces an increase in the quantity demanded until a new equilibrium is reached. To some extent this mechanism may also be operative in the market for physicians' services. Part of the "cost" of using a physician is the time and trouble involved in making an appointment, getting to his office, waiting, and the like. As the supply increases, this part of the cost tends to decrease, thus encouraging additional use. We hypothesize that in this particular market another force is also at work, namely, the ability of the physician to directly influence the demand for his own services. The data we have examined cannot prove the validity of this hypothesis but are certainly consistent with it.

We know that there was a large increase in the rate of change in utilization during 1956-66 compared with 1948-56. We also know that there was a substantial independent increase in the rate of change in supply during the same period. The growth of utilization did not result from the downward pressure of supply on price (movement along the demand curve), nor can it be attributed to shifts in the demand curve as a result of differential changes in income, insurance, or demographic structure. It seems to us very plausible that, instead, it was partly attributable to a physician-induced growth in demand and partly to the technologically-inspired growth in demand discussed in the previous section.

1.9   Quantity per Physician

The preceding discussion of changes in quantity of physicians' services per capita and number of physicians per capita makes it apparent that the quantity of service produced by each physician was not static during the period under study. The purpose of this section is to identify the various elements that contributed to the change in quantity per physician. Unfortunately, a paucity of reliable data on number of visits per physician makes it impossible to carry out this analysis for the subperiods.

We see in Table 14 that between 1948 and 1968 quantity per physician grew at an average annual rate of 2.1 per cent. This increase was not attributable in any measure to a larger number of visits per physician. In fact, the number of visits per physician seems to have declined slightly. What we observe is, rather, a considerable increase in the quantity of service supplied per visit.

This increase of 2.8 per cent per annum can be explained in part by the growth of specialization. It is well established that specialists have higher average receipts per visit than general practitioners (albeit they have fewer visits per week). The higher receipts per visit are the result of three factors. First, most specialists charge more for their own time than most general practitioners. Second, a visit to a specialist often involves more physician time. Finally, a visit to a specialist

TABLE 14

Statistical Analysis of Rate of Change in Quantity of Service per Physician, 1948-68

	Average Annual Rate of Change, per cent 1948-68
Quantity per physician	2.1
Visits per physician	-0.7
Quantity per visit	2.8
Shift to specialists[a,b]	0.9
Quantity per visit adjusted for shift to specialists.	1.9

Note: Rate of change of number of physicians based on 1949-67.

Source: See Appendix A and Tables 1, 3, 12, and 13.

[a] Based on change in distribution of visits between general practitioners and specialists and ratio of receipts for each type of visit.
[b] 1947-66 growth rate.

usually is accompanied by more auxiliary services, such as electrocardiograms, blood tests, and x-rays. On the basis of statistics published in *Medical Economics*, we have calculated that the average visit to a specialist results in nearly twice as much total expenditure (physician receipts) as the average visit to a G.P. ($10.55 versus $5.48 in 1966). A routine office visit to a specialist results in an expenditure of about 50 per cent more than a routine office visit to a G.P., ($6.35 versus $4.31 in 1966), and the cost of supplementary care received during an average visit to a specialist is about 260 per cent greater than that provided during a G.P. visit.[14]

As the percentage of physicians who are specialists grows, it is natural to expect some increase in quantity per visit. Furthermore, the last line of Table 14 shows that even after the shift towards specialization is taken into account, a substantial increase remains, which

---

[14] The *Medical Economics* statistics employed in these calculations pertain to annual gross receipts, visits per week, weeks worked per year, and standard fees for the routine office visits, for G.P.'s and for most categories of specialists. Multiplying the standard fee charged by the 1966 ratio of average price to customary price yields an average receipts figure for the routine office visit.

probably reflects the increased use of tests, x-rays, and other procedures by physicians of both types.

1.10 Analysis of Average Price

It has been shown that a large part of the increase in expenditures per capita is attributable to the increase in average price. In Table 15 we present a statistical analysis of some of the factors that might explain this price rise.

The most obvious explanatory variable is the rise in the general price level. Other things being equal, there is no reason to expect physicians' prices to remain stagnant while the rest of the economy is experiencing inflation. We see that the changes in the general price level, as measured by the Consumer Price Index, do explain part of the increase in the price of physicians' services, but neither for the subperiods nor for the period as a whole do they explain even as much as half of the increase.

A second major explanatory variable is differential movements in productivity. A widely accepted general-

ization in economics is that sectors with relatively low rates of growth of output per man have relatively rapid increases in price, and vice versa. For the nine major sectors of the economy the rank correlation between changes in price and changes in output per man, 1947-65, was −0.93 [18]. The reason for this is that compensation for the factors of production must, in the long run, increase at about the same rate in all sectors. Those with slow productivity growth need rapid price increases in order to generate enough revenue to pay for the capital and labor they employ. Conversely, if an industry or sector with rapid productivity growth did not have a slow growth of prices (or a decline), very large profits would be generated; new competitors would be attracted to the industry and existing ones would try to expand output, and the resulting increase in supply would tend to drive prices down.

The differential change in productivity here is estimated by comparing quantity per physician with real gross national product per person engaged.[15] For the period as a whole, productivity in the total economy rose somewhat faster than in the physician sector (2.5 per cent versus 2.1 per cent per annum), but after taking this into account we still find an unexplained rise in average price of physicians' services of 2.1 per cent per annum.

The size of the unexplained excess rise in average price varies considerably among the subperiods. During 1948-56, movements in the general price level and the differential in productivity explain nearly all of the rise in average price. The excess is much greater in 1956-66, and greater still in 1966-68.

The excess rise in the price of physicians' services implies that physicians were probably improving their relative income position. Some fragmentary data lend support to this conclusion. According to *Medical Economics*, the median net income of physicians from self-employment practice rose 17 per cent from 1966 to 1968. IRS data show a rise in average net business receipts per physician of 19 per cent during that two-year span.

1.11 The 1966-68 Subperiod

The years since 1966 have witnessed an extremely rapid rise in expenditures for physicians' services.

TABLE 15

Statistical Analysis of Rate of Change in Average Price of
Physicians' Services, 1948-68

(per cent per annum)

	1948-56	1956-66	1966-68	1948-68
Average price......	4.4	3.6	8.1	4.2
CPI, all goods and services	1.8	1.5	3.5	1.7
Excess of average price over general price level	2.6	2.1	4.6	2.5
Differential change in productivity[a]	1.7	0.4	0.6	0.4
Unexplained rise in average price	0.9	1.7	4.0	2.1

Source: See Appendix A and Tables 4 and 14.

[a] Differential change in productivity is derived as follows:

	1948-56	1956-66	1966-68	1948-68
Real GNP per person engaged	2.7	2.8	1.3	2.5
Minus: quantity per physician	1.0	2.4	0.7	2.1
Equals: differential change in productivity	1.7	0.4	0.6	0.4

---

[15] "Persons engaged" is a measure of all employed and self-employed persons in the United States adjusted to a full-time equivalent basis.

Because of the short time span, the paucity of data, and the likelihood that some of the data now available will be revised, a full-scale attempt to analyze this subperiod is not yet warranted. We do feel obliged, however, to call attention to some major departures in recent years from the trends of 1956-66, and to suggest a few tentative explanations.

The first major point to be noted about 1966-68 compared with the preceding decade is that the increase in average price was extremely rapid and accounted for almost all of the increase in per capita expenditures. Whereas quantity per capita had been rising at an average annual rate of 3.0 per cent, the rate of growth fell to 0.9 per cent in 1966-68. The rapid growth of third-party payments during this period meant that the net price to the patient declined relative to other prices; we might, therefore, have expected a rise in the quantity demanded on that account. Trends in income and age-sex structure also were in the direction of increasing demand.

Assuming that the figures are correct, we can see that there was a sharp falling off in the growth rate of quantity per physician from 1966 to 1968. One plausible explanation for the simultaneous sharp decrease in the growth rate of utilization may have been a weakened incentive on the part of physicians to actively cultivate a market for their services in the face of rapid price increases (8.1 per cent per annum as opposed to 3.6 per cent during the previous decade). Such a diminution in physician-induced demand growth is what we would expect with a supply function negatively related to average price, i.e., a backward-bending supply curve. In other words, the advent of Medicare and Medicaid produced a sharp increase in demand; physicians responded by raising their prices. This price increase, far from inducing physicians to work more, made it possible for them to earn higher incomes while actually working less.

The speculative nature of this account must be emphasized; in order to make a more definitive analysis we need more data and a longer time period for study. Statistics on hours and weeks worked by each physician would be particularly helpful. Also, it should be noted that the increased paperwork associated with third-party payment may have been partly responsible for the relative stagnation in quantity per physician. It does seem likely, however, that the vast sums of money poured into physicians' services by the government in recent years served to increase the incomes of physicians (and possibly to redistribute their services) rather than to call forth an increase in overall quantity of their services. To the extent that physicians were already working up to their capacity in 1966, this result was almost inevitable, since the supply of physicians responds, if at all, only after a long lag.

2
Differences Across States, 1966:
An Econometric Analysis

2.1 Introduction

Part 1 has suggested the importance of advances in medical technology in explaining postwar trends in expenditures, utilization, and physician productivity. In order to gain an understanding of physician and patient behavior net of technological change, we now turn to a cross-sectional model. By examining differences across states at a single point in time we are in effect holding medical technology fairly constant. There may be some lag in the spread of new knowledge from one state to another, but the difference between the frontier of knowledge in the most and least advanced states in any given year is far less than the change that occurred between 1948 and 1968 in the United States as a whole.[1]

Another advantage of the cross-sectional approach is that it provides an opportunity to learn something about the factors influencing the supply of physicians. It is widely recognized that there are substantial barriers to entry into medicine. These are partly financial and partly caused by the reluctance of organized medicine to expand the volume of training facilities to the point where all applicants with an ability to pay would be accepted. Moreover, it takes a long time to establish a new medical school, and there is a lag of five or more years between the time a student enters medical school and the time he begins to practice. It follows that the total number of practicing physicians in the country cannot be responsive to any important degree to annual changes in price or other market conditions. By contrast, the potential elasticity of physician supply going to any one state is very great. Previous investigators have already demonstrated that licensing procedures pose no significant impediment to interstate migration of physi-

cians. (See [7], [24].) With entry into the total market effectively limited, the geographical distribution of physicians has become a matter of particular concern.

2.2 A Framework for Analysis

Per capita expenditures for physicians' services vary considerably across states. In 1966, such expenditures were $68.68 in California compared with $26.42 in South Carolina.[2] This is a greater variation than the change that occurred in the national average between 1948 and 1965.

How are we to explain such large variations in expenditures? By definition, expenditures are equal to quantity multiplied by price. More fundamentally, then, our task is to explain interstate variations in price and quantity. To do this economists employ a general model of demand and supply. In such a model the quantity demanded by consumers depends upon price and many other variables, some of which are applicable to any commodity, e.g., per capita income, and others that may be relevant only to one or a few commodities, e.g., health insurance. The quantity provided by suppliers is also treated as a function of price and other variables. In equilibrium, the quantity demanded is exactly equal to the quantity supplied; hence, actual quantity and actual price are simultaneously determined through the interaction of the demand and supply functions.

Specification of a model for physicians' services establishes a general framework within which a broad range of hypotheses regarding the behavior of patients and physicians can be investigated. Each structural equation of the model offers an explanation for the determinants of a particular aspect of the market for

---

[1] Differences in actual medical practice across states are undoubtedly larger than differences in the frontier of medical knowledge. Our interpretation of the technological factor in demand, however, is predicated upon the assumption that the demand for physicians' services increases with an expansion in the range of services physicians are *technically* able to offer. Variations in actual medical practice across states are viewed primarily as the consequence of variations in demand rather than as their cause.

[2] The range of variation in per capita disposable income was substantially less in that year for the thirty-three states in our sample, having a high value of $3,185 in Connecticut and a low of $1,586 in Mississippi. The coefficients of variation for per capita physician expenditures and per capita income were 24.0 per cent and 16.0 per cent, respectively. State data for 1965 and 1967 show about the same degree of variation as in 1966.

physicians' services. Our model has one equation dealing with variations in demand, one for the number of physicians, one for physician productivity, and one for the amount of insurance coverage.

Because the variables we wish to explain are not determined independently of one another, it is not possible to test our behavioral hypotheses accurately with ordinary least-squares regression equations. For example, one clear implication of the interdependency among these variables is that we cannot discover the true influence of price on physicians' locational choice by simply relating the total number of physicians practicing in a state to the observed price of physicians' services there. Possibly a demand-induced rise in price does tend to attract many physicians to a state; but this increase in supply will serve to depress price back towards its original level if the population can only be induced to purchase the additional services at a somewhat reduced price.

To cope with this problem we estimate each of the structural equations of our model by means of two-stage least squares. This procedure allows one to statistically disentangle the web of mutual causality in order to isolate the specific effect of one variable on another. The method consists of obtaining predicted values for each endogenous variable by regressing it on all of the exogenous variables in the model.[3] This is the first stage. The structural equation for each endogenous variable is then estimated by regressing the actual value of that variable on the predicted values of appropriate endogenous variables and on relevant exogenous variables. This is the second stage. With endogenous variables represented by their predicted values, the estimated regression coefficients are not biased by any effect that the dependent variables may have on them.

When employing this two-stage procedure for estimating relationships involving simultaneously determined variables, *only those exogenous variables that appear in the model should be used in estimation of the first stage.* Use of any other exogenous variables may improve the fit in a given sample, but this improvement is spurious because the additional variables play no independent role in the system. A priori considerations can suggest which variables, endogenous and exogenous, are potentially important in explaining the variation we

observe, but the final determination of which variables to include in the model is itself an empirical question. Once experimentation with a preliminary, large-scale model determines that certain exogenous variables are actually of no value in the second-stage equations, a new set of first-stage endogenous variable estimates should be formed, based only on the more restricted set of exogenous variables that have been shown to bear a significant relation to the supply-demand mechanism.[4] The rejected hypotheses of the initial model are, of course, an integral part of the conclusions of such an analysis.

The model we present in the following section excludes many variables that one might reasonably expect to affect the demand for, or supply of, physicians' services. The reason for their omission is that tests based upon a preliminary model employing seventeen exogenous variables revealed that only five of these did, in fact, appear in the system.[5] On these grounds we excluded the other twelve exogenous variables from the condensed version of the model presented below, which alone can be considered to possess an unbiased set of first-stage (predicted) endogenous variables. Discussions of the excluded variables and their role in the original model are incorporated into section 2.3, under the appropriate subheadings. A complete list of the variables appearing in each model is presented in Table 16.

2.3 Specification of the Model

The interrelationships among the six endogenous and five exogenous variables of our final model can be summarized by four structural equations and two identities:[6]

$$(1) \quad Q^*_D = Q^*_D (\hat{AP} \text{ or } \hat{NP}, \hat{BEN}^*, \hat{MD}^*, INC^*, BEDS^*).$$

$$(2) \quad MD^* = MD^* (\hat{AP}, \hat{Q/MD}, MED\ SCLS, BEDS^*, INC^*).$$

---

[3] Endogenous variables are determined within the system ("jointly determined"), while exogenous variables are determined outside the system ("predetermined").

[4] We are indebted to Christopher Sims of the National Bureau for bringing this to our attention.

[5] Some of the excluded exogenous variables were significant in equations in which they appeared, e.g., race as a determinant of health status, but because the endogenous variable health was found to be insignificant in the demand equation, both health and race factored out of the system.

[6] The circumflex (∧) over a variable indicates that its predicted value is used in estimating the equation. An asterisk (*) indicates that the variable is phrased in per capita terms.

TABLE 16

List of Variables

Final Model	Preliminary Model	Full Title of Variable (Units)
		Endogenous
Q*	Q*	Quantity per capita (visits)[a]
MD*	MD*	Private physicians per 100,000 population
Q/MD	Q/MD	Quantity per private physician (visits)[a]
AP	AP	Average price (dollars)
BEN*	BEN*	Insurance benefits per capita (dollars)
NP	NP	Net price (dollars)
	INF MRT	Infant mortality rate per 1,000 live births
	DTH RT	Crude death rate per 1,000 population
		Exogenous
INC*	INC*	Disposable personal income per capita (dollars)
BEDS*	BEDS*	Short-term hospital beds per 1,000 population
MED SCLS	MED SCLS	Number of medical schools
PRM/BEN	PRM/BEN	Ratio of health insurance premiums to benefits
UNION*	UNION*	Union members per 100 population
	EDUC	Median years of education, persons 25 and over
	%BLK	Per cent black
	%AGED	Per cent 65 and over
	%URB	Per cent urban
	BRTH RT	Births per 1,000 population
	TEMP	Mean temperature, average of major cities (degrees F.)
	S&L GOV*	State and local government expenditures for health per capita (dollars)
	HOSP MD*	Hospital staff physicians per 100,000 population
	ΔINC*	Change in disposable personal income per capita 1960-66 (dollars)
	%PART	Per cent of private physicians in partnership practice
	%SPEC	Per cent of private physicians who are specialists
	MD ORIG*	Physicians originating per 100,000 population[b]

[a] G.P. outpatient visit equivalents.
[b] Total of six sample years.

$$(3) \quad Q/MD = Q/MD \, (\hat{AP}, \hat{MD}, BEDS*).$$

$$(4) \quad BEN* = BEN* \, (\hat{Q}*, \hat{AP}, UNIONS*, PRM/BEN, INC*).$$

$$(5) \quad Q*_D \equiv (MD*) \, (Q/MD) \equiv Q*_S.$$

$$(6) \quad NP \equiv \frac{\text{Expenditures} - \text{Benefits}}{\text{Expenditures}} (AP)$$

$$\equiv \frac{AP \cdot Q* - BEN*}{AP \cdot Q*} (AP).$$

These relationships are presented diagrammatically in Figures 1 and 2.

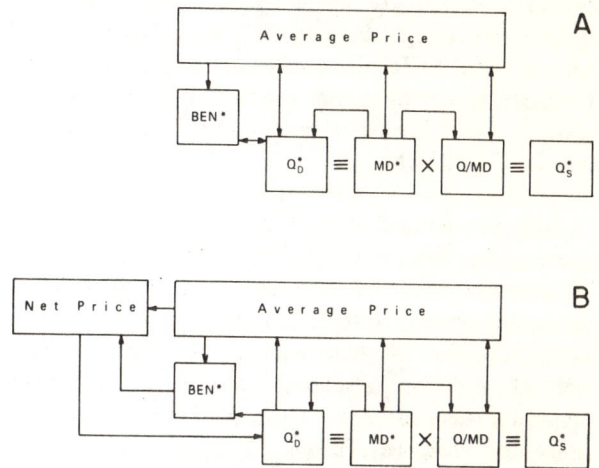

Figure 1.—Relationships Among Endogenous Variables, Alternate Specifications

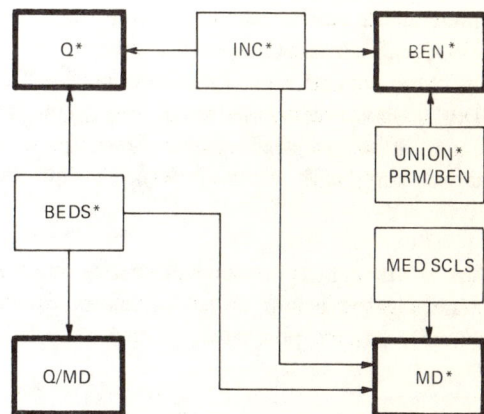

Figure 2.—Effects of Exogenous Variables on Endogenous Variables

In this equilibrium model of the market for physicians' services, the quantity of service demanded per capita (Q^*_D) is identically equal to the product of the two supply variables, number of physicians per capita (MD*) and quantity of service per physician (Q/MD).[7] Because it seems unreasonable to suppose that purchases of medical insurance are unrelated to the price and quantity of the physicians' services covered, medical insurance benefits appear endogenously in the model. Price is represented by two variables: the average price received by physicians for their services (AP) and the net price paid by consumers (NP), which AP exceeds according to the degree to which insurance benefits pay for the cost of the average visit. AP and NP are thus comparable to the time series variables of the same name discussed in Part 1. The exogenous variables in this system are per capita income (INC*), number of medical schools (MED SCLS), hospital beds per capita (BEDS*), labor union members per capita (UNION*), and the ratio of health insurance premiums to health insurance benefits (PRM/BEN).

Both the demand for and the supply of physicians' services are thought to be subject to special forces. Whenever possible, we have attempted to incorporate the unique features often attributed to this market into our model. The following equation-by-equation discussion of the four structural equations listed above considers these issues and indicates the range of questions that can be illuminated by a cross-sectional analysis.

Demand (Q^*_D)

Prices and income are the customary economic determinants of market demand. How important are these financial considerations to consumers in determining their demand for physicians' services? Is the quantity of service demanded at all sensitive to its own price, and if so, to what extent? Does the quantity demanded vary with income? What is the income elasticity?

What is the role of medical insurance in demand? Some investigators believe that it is a major influence on the quantity of care purchased, yet our analysis of the

time series data yields no evidence indicative of a systematic relationship between changes in benefit levels and changes in Q*.

A related question concerns the mechanism by which insurance operates on demand (if, indeed, it does). In one specification of the model, NP replaces AP as the relevant demand price variable. The argument for so doing is that the impact of insurance can be entirely attributed to the reduction it effects in the net price of care. The substitution of NP for AP also implies that patients are indifferent to variations in the average amount collected by physicians so long as they are not personally responsible for financing the differentials. A less restrictive test of the role of insurance in demand retains AP as the price variable and adds to the equation the benefits variable, BEN*. This specification leaves open the manner in which insurance affects demand. It also allows for the possibility that consumers are influenced even by those variations in AP which do not translate into variations in NP. If price-consciousness is a firmly ingrained consumer trait, changes in the institutional arrangements governing a particular market may not be strong enough to suppress altogether the usual behavior mechanism whereby low cost goods and services are sought out, regardless of who gets the bill.

Certain services provided by private practice physicians can only be consumed in hospitals: intensive diagnostic work-ups and most surgical procedures are common examples. To a limited extent, then, the services offered by hospitals and by private practice physicians constitute a joint consumption product, hospitalized medical care. If for any reason the supply of hospital beds influences the quantity of hospital care people purchase, an increase in BEDS* may affect the demand for physicians' services as well.

The market for physicians' services is characterized by a high degree of consumer ignorance concerning the need for services and the central role of the physician as an authoritative advisor regarding their use. Given these circumstances, we hypothesize that physicians are able to *generate* a demand for their services without lowering price; we therefore include MD* in the demand equation. When physicians are abundant in a state, they may order care which is not medically indicated (e.g., unnecessary surgery) or of only marginal importance (e.g., cosmetic procedures, numerous postoperative visits, overzealous well-baby care). Alternatively, when physicians are very scarce, patients may lower their

---

[7] It would, of course, be possible to combine the two dimensions of supply into one overall supply equation, but to do so would be to discard much valuable information regarding the behavior of physicians.

expectations and handle minor complaints with a minimum of physician intervention. There is also another reason why the supply of physicians might exercise a direct influence on the demand for physicians' services. A significant part of the cost incurred by the patient is in the form of time spent in travel and in waiting rooms. A reduction in the relative scarcity of physicians is usually associated with both an improvement in their locational distribution and a decrease in waiting room time. To the extent that the ease or difficulty of seeing a physician is a determinant of demand, we have a second justification for including MD* in the demand equation.

The independent variables in our demand equation thus fall into two categories: economic variables common to any demand analysis (price, income) and institutional factors peculiar to this market (insurance, hospital bed supply, physician supply). Ten additional variables—most of which fall under the heading of "taste" factors—were tested in the preliminary version of the model (see section 2.2). Because none proved to be statistically significant or measurably improved the fit of the equations, these were omitted from the final version of the model presented here, inasmuch as their inclusion would have injected a bias into the first-stage endogenous variable estimates. The rejected demand variables are: education (median years of school of persons 25 and over), urbanization, two measures of health status (the infant mortality rate and the crude death rate), per cent black, per cent aged, the birth rate, mean annual temperature, per capita state and local government expenditures for physicians' services, and number of hospital staff physicians per capita. The last two variables attempted to measure the availability of alternative sources of supply of physicians' services (services by physicians other than private practitioners, who alone enter our study).

Supply of Physicians (MD*)

It is hypothesized that one variable influencing physician location is price. AP is clearly the relevant supply price variable, since it is of little import to the physician whether payment originates with his patients or with insurance companies.[8] To what extent is the

present level of inequality in the distribution of physicians—the number of private practitioners per 100,000 ranges from sixty in Mississippi to 134 in New York—attributable to differences in price?

With price held constant, per capita income serves as a taste factor in this equation. Specifically, INC* is here a proxy for the level of cultural, educational, social, and recreational opportunities which a state has to offer. Because physicians as a group are very high earners, nonpecuniary factors of this sort may be a major consideration in their location decision.

Another possible influence on physician distribution is the quality and availability of complementary medical facilities. As a test of this hypothesis we include MED SCLS and BEDS* in the MD* supply equation.

Finally, we investigate the possibility that physicians are disinclined to open a practice in states where the average workload of their would-be colleagues is high. We should observe a negative sign on the endogenous variable Q/MD if it is true that physicians shun areas where they might feel under pressure to work long hours and/or spend less time per patient than they deem optimal.

Originally, we hypothesized that physicians would show some partiality toward their state of origin prior to entry into medical school, but tests with this variable in the preliminary model led to its rejection. Also, no support was found for the view that physicians are drawn to practice in the medically neediest states, with medical need being measured by infant mortality (an endogenous variable), and therefore health, too, was excluded from this equation in the final model.

Quantity of Service per Physician (Q/MD)

The real quantity of services provided by individual physicians varies considerably across states, the coefficient of variation being 15.4 per cent. These productivity differences are an important factor in the interstate variations in physician gross income, which are quite large in view of the fairly high uniformity of skill among physicians.

Three factors are considered as possible influences on physician productivity. As with the supply variable, the relationship with price is an important matter to investigate. Do physicians respond to higher prices by

---

[8] Physician behavior might conceivably be affected if the source of payment were governmental, because of the consequent red tape and the physician's personal political philosophy. However, only private insurance is considered in this analysis; data on governmental expenditures for physicians' services are unavailable on a state basis.

working more hours and by seeing more patients per hour, or do they display a backward-bending supply curve, cutting back on their workload and maintaining their income while gaining the benefits of additional leisure and a less hectic pace of activity?

An increase in the supply of hospital beds should raise Q/MD if physicians have a tendency to hospitalize more readily whenever the necessary facilities are available.[9] This behavior might arise if there is a technological imperative on the part of physicians to practice the most up-to-date medicine within their grasp.

One of the most critical matters to be investigated is whether areas with a relative scarcity of physicians are partly relieved by enjoying higher physician productivity. It is our hypothesis that the average physician, because of the nature of his professional training, feels under some ethical and social compulsion to supply additional services, even at the same rate of remuneration, when he is in an area poorly endowed with physicians. Thus, we anticipate a negative sign on the $\hat{MD}$* variable in the Q/MD equation.

Two other variables were initially tested in this regression: the degree of physician specialization and the extent of partnership (as opposed to solo proprietorship) practice. As neither proved to be significant, the two were omitted from the final model now under consideration.

Insurance (BEN*)

The argument for treating insurance as an endogenous phenomenon can be made on two grounds. The first is that the amount of insurance purchased depends upon the expected level of outlays people are insuring against. Assuming a generally risk-averse population, an increase in expected outlays should call forth the purchase of additional insurance protection. Expected outlays will be highly dependent upon expenditures in the recent past, and the best proxy for this in our model is expenditures in the present. The predicted values of both expenditure components, price and quantity, appear as explanatory variables in the insurance equation as a test of this hypothesis. If it is correct, the estimated coefficients of both variables should be (approximately)

equal when the regressions are estimated in double-logarithmic form. If risk aversion itself rises (is constant, or falls) with the level of expected loss, the coefficients will exceed (equal, or fall short of) 1.0.

The other rationale for regarding insurance as endogenous lays stress on the cost of insurance itself rather than on the perceived need for the financial protection it offers. The cost of insurance is defined by the relation PIV = (PRM/BEN) (AP) − AP. PRM/BEN is the ratio of health insurance premiums to benefits, i.e., the average price of purchasing one dollar of health insurance benefits (a figure greater than one). PIV thus represents the average price of insuring one G.P. visit equivalent over and above the price of purchasing it directly. The reason for carrying insurance is that, in the event of extraordinary medical expenses, the return to an individual who expends PRM/BEN will be many times greater than one. Of course, there is also the inherent chance that the return will be as low as zero, but that is the gamble an insured person takes. On the average, an insurance payment of PIV is the nonrecoverable price one pays to be reimbursed for one G.P. visit equivalent. The cost of insuring a given number of visits is thus seen to depend on two factors, the "fairness" of insurance policies and the price of physicians' services.

PRM/BEN is exogenous in our model, being dependent upon such factors as the extent of group coverage compared with individual coverage, and the relative importance of policies issued by nonprofit insuring organizations such as Blue Shield. AP, by contrast, is endogenous. If PIV is found to influence the consumer's willingness to insure, insurance itself is endogenous as a result of this dependence. Because PIV is the price of insuring one visit equivalent and not the price of a dollar's worth of insurance benefits, the dependent variable in this specification should really be the number of insured visit equivalents, or BEN*/AP. For consistency with the financial protection theory of insurance, which demands a dollar measure of benefits, we maintain the BEN* form throughout. When we wish to interpret the price coefficient as the price elasticity of demand for insured visits, however, we must first subtract 1.0 from its estimated value.

In addition to PRM/BEN, two other exogenous variables enter the insurance function: per capita income and the degree of unionization. The potential effectiveness of unions derives from their role in winning fringe benefits in the form of health insurance policies (particu-

---

[9] Our measure of physician output weights hospital inpatient visits higher than outpatient visits because of differences in their relative prices.

larly desirable because of their untaxed status). Unionization should raise the percentage of the population covered by insurance, since the decision to insure is no longer left to the discretion of the individual, and may also increase the mean level of benefits per insured.

In the preliminary version of our model we tested the hypothesis that people are differentially inclined to insure a newly acquired standard of living as compared to one which has been long held. The change in per capita income over the previous six years proved insignificant in the benefits equation, however, and so was dropped from the final list of exogenous variables. Also rejected on the basis of these early tests was the level of education as a determinant of BEN*.

2.4 The Data

The data used in this analysis come from a variety of sources and are of varying reliability. The critical expenditures and visit series regrettably are not of a kind in which we can place a high degree of confidence. Because interstate variations in these quantities are substantial and move in directions that remain fairly consistent from one year to the next, empirical analysis of the available data does seem justifiable. Nonetheless, until such time as a better data base has been established, conclusions derived from this study can only be suggestive of the true underlying relationships.

Expenditures

Our study population consists of the thirty-three states for which expenditures data are available for 1966.[10] Most of the omitted states have small populations; their absence does not have much effect on the results because each observation in our model is weighted by the square root of the state population. The thirty-three states accounted for 90 per cent of the total U.S. population. The expenditures data come from the Internal Revenue Service and represent the reported gross receipts from medical practice of all self-employed physicians. Thus, this series is comparable to the expenditures data examined in the section on time trends (Part 1).

Availability of expenditures data was one of the key factors in our selection of a year for the cross-sectional

analysis. As of this writing, state data on the gross business receipts of "offices of physicians and surgeons" have been published for only five other postwar years. With the exception of 1949 (for which these figures are obtainable for forty-eight states), the size of the sample has been limited (twenty-seven states for fiscal 1960-61, twenty-two for 1963, twenty-eight for 1965, and twenty-six for 1967). The other controlling factor in our decision was the availability of data on physician visits from the National Health Survey. The choice here was between 1957-59, 1963-64, and 1966-67. 1966 was chosen because the requisite expenditures data were available for a relatively large number of states and visit data were also specific to that year.

The accuracy of the expenditures series is not easy to check. The possibility of some underreporting of income is suggested by the fact that the IRS data imply average gross receipts per physician of $46,600, compared with a median of $49,000 reported in *Medical Economics* for the same year. On the other hand, at least some of this disparity is explainable by the fact that *Medical Economics* only surveys full-time, self-employed physicians under the age of sixty-five, while the IRS total includes the smaller average receipts of older physicians and of hospital staff and faculty physicians who devote just a fraction of their working time to private practice. Furthermore, only if the degree of underreporting varied significantly across states would this factor impair the validity of an analysis of variations in expenditures.

Far more serious is the distinct possibility that errors in this series are not uniform across states but have a sizable random component. Our suspicions on this count are based upon intertemporal correlations of expenditures per capita across the twenty-six states for which these data are available for 1965, 1966, and 1967. The correlation coefficient for the 1965-66 comparison is 0.863, and for 1966-67, 0.912.[11] While these figures are high enough to show that there is *something* systematic worth investigating in the pattern of variation in 1966 expenditures, they compare unfavorably with the (weighted) correlation coefficients for per capita disposable income in these states from one year to the next: 0.998 for 1965-66 and 0.997 for 1966-67. Closer examination of the official expenditures data reveals that states with the most extreme jumps in expenditures had parallel shifts in the number of physicians said to be

---

[10] All series refer to 1966 unless otherwise indicated.

[11] These correlations are weighted by 1966 state population. The unweighted correlations are 0.760 and 0.824, respectively.

filing business income tax returns. These reported shifts in the number of physicians filing returns show virtually no correspondence to changes in the number of physicians practicing in each state, a statistical series kept by the American Medical Association.[12] To cite two of the most extreme examples, the IRS figures show a gain of 45.1 per cent from 1966 to 1967 in the number of physicians filing returns in Wisconsin, and a fall of 25.8 per cent in the number filing in Louisiana. According to the AMA, however, the number of practicing physicians in these two states rose by 1.2 per cent and 2.0 per cent, respectively, over this period.[13] It is apparent that official statistics on health care expenditures are in much need of improvement. Changes in nationwide expenditures totals over long periods no doubt provide a fairly accurate indication of changes actually taking place. For specific years or specific states, however, deficiencies in the statistical data now constitute a major impediment to serious research.

Physicians

The scope of the market for physicians' services relevant to our study does not extend beyond the

---

[12] Simple regressions across states of the annual change in total expenditures $\frac{EXP_{t+1}}{EXP_t}$ on the annual change in physicians filing returns $\frac{IRS_{t+1}}{IRS_t}$ show the independent variable to be highly significant and the explanatory power of the equation fairly high. $\frac{IRS_{t+1}}{IRS_t}$, however, bears almost no relation to the percentage change in private practitioners $\frac{MD_{t+1}}{MD_t}$, as recorded by the AMA, even though the correlation between IRS and MD for any given year is on the order of .99.

Dependent Variable	Independent Variable	Coefficient (Standard Error)	R^2
$\frac{EXP_{67}}{EXP_{66}}$	$\frac{IRS_{67}}{IRS_{66}}$	.50 (.13)	.40
$\frac{EXP_{66}}{EXP_{65}}$	$\frac{IRS_{66}}{IRS_{65}}$	.66 (.10)	.63
$\frac{IRS_{67}}{IRS_{66}}$	$\frac{MD_{67}}{MD_{66}}$	1.82 (1.99)	.03
$\frac{IRS_{66}}{IRS_{65}}$	$\frac{MD_{66}}{MD_{65}}$	1.09 (2.69)	.01

[13] The AMA figures refer to private practice physicians only.

bounds of private practice. As the official expenditures series is limited to physicians' gross receipts from self-employment practice, so the MD series we have chosen (our source is the American Medical Association) is restricted to private practitioners.

Unlike the IRS count of physicians filing business income tax returns, the AMA data have the conceptual advantage of including salaried physicians in private practice, whose services go to meet the same demand as those of the self-employed and whose contribution to gross receipts may be considerable. The fact that the AMA bases its count on the results of routine questionnaires sent annually to all physicians while the IRS estimate derives from a sample of physicians filing a rather unpopular tax report makes the AMA series superior from a statistical viewpoint. Also, as noted above, the extreme instability of the IRS figures calls into question that data-gathering process itself. Unfortunately, neither the AMA nor the IRS series permits us to calculate precisely the number of full-time equivalent physicians in private practice; the former covers physicians whose *principal* mode of employment is private practice, while the latter covers all physicians with some self-employment income, no matter how small a fraction of their professional time is involved. On balance, however, the AMA series probably more closely approximates the desired figure of full-time equivalent physicians, since it includes some but not all part-timers and since it is not restricted to the self-employed.

Quantity and Average Price

Two of the most important series, quantity of service and average price, are not directly available and must be estimated. The quantity series we estimate is a measure of "general practitioner (G. P.) outpatient visit equivalents," a fairly homogeneous unit across states. Dividing expenditures by quantity then gives us an implicit price series, which represents the average price of a G. P. outpatient visit equivalent.

The quantity series is derived in the following way. The National Center for Health Statistics has published data on home and office visits per capita for the four census regions in 1966-67 and for the nine census divisions in 1957-59. We assume an intraregion per capita visit distribution of the 1966-67 data based on the distribution that prevailed in the earlier period. The resulting home and office visit figure for each division is then attributed to each state within that division.

Next, the number of hospital visits is estimated for each state from the number of patient days spent in nonfederal short-term hospitals. Our assumption of one visit for each day of stay is supported by *Medical Economics*, which reports that the median number of hospital visits made by private practitioners in 1966 was twenty-two per week and that the median number of weeks worked per year was forty-eight. If private practitioners in the thirty-three states of our study conformed to the *Medical Economics* medians, they would have made 177 million hospital visits. In fact, the total number of patient days in these states was very close to this, 185 million. Combining these disparate visit series, hospital inpatient visits are given a weight of 1.71 relative to home and office visits, this being the national ratio of average charges for the two categories of visits, according to Department of Health, Education, and Welfare statistics.[14]

A final adjustment takes account of the fact that the distribution of total visits between G. P.'s and specialists varies across states. A visit to a specialist is accorded a weight of 1.93 relative to a G. P. visit, based on the ratio of average gross receipts per visit. In estimating the percentage of total visits made by specialists in each state, we, of course, make an allowance for the smaller visit load of specialists (.63 as many visits as G. P.'s).[15]

There undoubtedly are some errors in the resulting quantity series and the price series derived from it, but we are not aware of any systematic biases. Some confirmation of the validity of the overall approach may be found in the fact that the resulting average price for a G. P. visit in our series is $5.75, which is very close to the $5.48 implicit in *Medical Economics* data for the same year.

Other Variables

All series pertaining to insurance are based upon data in the *Source Book of Health Insurance*, an annual publication of the Health Insurance Institute. The two endogenous insurance variables, BEN* and NP, refer only to insurance coverage for physicians' services, i.e., surgical, regular medical, and a share of major medical.

The exogenous PRM/BEN variable pertains to all forms of health insurance (physician, hospital, and disability).

Information regarding the number of medical schools in each state (MED SCLS) is taken from the annual education issue of the *Journal of the American Medical Association*. BEDS* represents the bed capacity of short-term, general, and other special hospitals, a series made available by the American Hospital Association. Figures on per capita disposable personal income in each state (INC*) are published in the *Survey of Current Business*. The *Statistical Abstract of the United States* provides data on labor union membership (UNION*).

Summary statistics for all variables are presented in Table 17. A complete description of the method developed to estimate Q* and the details of all other calculations may be found in Appendix C, which also includes specific source references, data tables listing the most important series, and a correlation matrix.

2.5 Regression Results

Table 18 presents the results of the second-stage regressions. All of the equations are estimated in double-logarithmic form, the estimated coefficients thus representing elasticities.[16] To avoid problems of heteroscedasticity, each observation is weighted by the square root of the state's population.[17] In computing the *t* statistics for each variable, we have made those adjustments appropriate for two-stage estimation.[18]

---

[14] Office of Research and Statistics, Social Security Administration, U.S. Department of Health, Education, and Welfare, "Current Medicare Survey Report," *Health Insurance Statistics*, CMS-12, January 27, 1970.

[15] Both figures are derived from survey data published in *Medical Economics* (see Appendix C).

[16] The one exception applies to MED SCLS, which is phrased as a linear variable because it sometimes takes on the value zero.

[17] Plots of the residuals from unweighted regressions demonstrate an inverse relationship between population and the size of the unexplained residual.

[18] *t* statistics are ordinarily obtained by dividing each coefficient by its standard error, but this procedure is not valid when the predicted values of endogenous variables appear on the right-hand side of an equation. In such cases the following adjustment is necessary: (1) Recompute the residuals for each observation by applying the estimated second-stage regression coefficients to the *actual* values of the included endogenous variables. (2) Obtain the ratio of the sum of squared residuals from the recomputed equation to the sum of squared residuals from the estimated regression. (3) Multiply each of the original *t* statistics for a particular regression equation by this factor (which may be equal to, greater than, or less than, 1.0) in order to arrive at a set of adjusted *t* statistics applicable to the second-stage regression. We are most grateful to Christopher Sims for bringing this to our attention.

TABLE 17

Summary Statistics, Thirty-three States, 1966

Symbol	Full Title of Variable (Units)	Mean[a]	Standard Deviation[a]	Coefficient of Variation (Per Cent)
EXP*	Expenditures per capita (dollars)	44.49	10.66	24.0
Q*	Quantity per capita (visits)[b]	7.71	.72	9.4
AP	Average price (dollars)	5.75	1.16	20.1
NP	Net price (dollars)	3.70	1.16	31.4
BEN*	Insurance benefits per capita (dollars)	16.00	4.29	26.8
MD*	Private physicians per 100,000 population	95.4	22.6	23.6
EXP/MD	Expenditures (gross income) per private physician (dollars)	47,003	5,900	12.6
Q/MD	Quantity per private physician (visits)[b]	8,354	1,290	15.4
DTH RT	Crude death rate per 1,000 population	9.42	.93	9.9
INF MRT	Infant mortality rate per 1,000 live births	23.7	3.2	13.6
INC*	Disposable personal income per capita (dollars)	2,605	418	16.0
MED SCLS	Number of medical schools	3.62	2.82	77.9
UNION*	Union members per 100 population	9.5	4.0	42.4
BEDS*	Short-term hospital beds per 1,000 population	3.78	.53	14.1
PRM/BEN	Ratio of health insurance premiums to benefits	1.27	.08	6.6
%SPEC	Per cent of private physicians who are specialists	64.9	5.9	9.0
ΔINC*	Change in disposable personal income per capita, 1960-66 (dollars)	663	89	13.4
EDUC	Median years of education, persons 25 & over	10.5	.98	9.3
%AGED	Per cent 65 and over	9.5	1.4	14.7
%BLK	Per cent black	11.2	8.7	78.3
%PART	Per cent of private physicians in partnership practice	24.1	8.6	35.5
BRTH RT	Birth rate per 1,000 population	18.5	1.17	6.3
MD ORIG*	Physicians originating per 1,000 population[c]	2.08	.61	29.4
S&L GOV*	State and local government expenditures for health, per capita (dollars)	34.26	11.41	33.3
HOSP MD*	Hospital staff physicians per 100,000 population	28.4	13.9	49.1
TEMP	Mean temperature, average of major cities (degrees F.)	56.3	7.1	12.5
%URB	Per cent urban	70.6	13.8	19.5

[a] Each observation weighted by square root of population of state.
[b] G. P. outpatient visits equivalents.
[c] Total of six sample years.

TABLE 18

Results of Weighted, Logarithmic Regressions, Second Stage, Interstate Model, 1966 (N=33)

Equation	$\bar{R}^2$	INC*	$\overset{\Lambda}{AP}$	$\overset{\Lambda}{NP}$	$\overset{\Lambda}{BEN*}$	$\overset{\Lambda}{MD*}$	BEDS*
			Part A: Q* (Quantity per Capita)				
A.1	.515	0.412[b] (5.92)					
A.2	.578	0.571[b] (9.25)	-0.290[b] (-3.58)				
A.3	.588	0.269 (1.64)	-0.205[a] (-2.25)		0.177 (1.99)		
A.4	.585		-0.104 (-1.65)		0.313[b] (9.97)		
A.5	.566	0.449[b] (9.94)		-0.153[b] (-3.24)			
A.6	.732	0.199[a] (2.54)	-0.356[b] (-5.28)			0.388[b] (6.28)	
A.7	.727	0.042 (0.61)		-0.200[b] (-5.55)		0.397[b] (6.90)	
A.8	.735			-0.201[b] (-5.63)		0.428[b] (15.10)	
A.9	.715		-0.297[b] (-4.16)			0.507[b] (11.22)	
A.10....	.746			-0.059 (-0.69)		0.359[b] (7.34)	0.193 (1.95)
A.11....	.752					0.335[b] (12.01)	0.252[b] (6.06)

Equation	$\bar{R}^2$	MED SCLS[c]	INC*	$\overset{\Lambda}{AP}$	BEDS*	$\overset{\Lambda}{Q/MD}$	
			Part B: MD* (Physicians per 100,000 Population)				
B.1	.521	0.059[b] (5.99)					
B.2	.754	0.036[b] (4.37)	0.750[b] (5.51)				
B.3	.731	0.050[b] (8.46)		0.828[b] (6.40)			
B.4	.509	0.061[b] (5.63)			-0.107 (-0.48)		
B.5	.775	0.040[b] (4.16)	0.490[a] (2.21)	0.419 (1.64)			
B.6	.784	0.036[b] (8.54)	0.071 (0.40)	1.052[b] (4.26)	0.492[b] (2.86)		

(Continued)

TABLE 18—Concluded

Equation	$\bar{R}^2$	MED SCLS[c]	INC*	$\hat{AP}$	BEDS*	$\hat{Q/MD}$
			Part B: MD* (Physicians per 100,000 Population)—Continued			
B.7......	.791	0.037^b (10.34)		1.144^b (14.64)	0.550^b (7.04)	
B.8......	.755	0.039^b (4.47)	0.759^b (5.57)		-0.161 (-1.02)	
B.9.	.783	0.032 (0.69)		0.994 (0.71)	0.528^a (2.35)	-0.199 (-0.11)
B.10.....	.776	0.027 (0.36)	0.080 (0.27)	0.752 (0.31)	0.443 (0.92)	-0.382 (-0.13)

Equation	$\bar{R}^2$	$\hat{AP}$	BEDS*	$\hat{MD}$	
		Part C: Q/MD (Quantity per Physician)			
C.1......	.420	-0.828^b (-3.84)			
C.2......	.603			-0.622^b (-3.25)	
C.3......	.622	-0.297 (-0.57)		-0.494 (-1.50)	
C.4......	.622	0.012 (0.01)	0.259 (0.39)	-0.672 (-1.21)	
C.5......	.635		0.252 (0.71)	-0.665^b (-2.80)	

Equation	$\bar{R}^2$	INC*	UNION*	PRM/BEN	$\hat{AP}$	$\hat{Q}*$
			Part D: BEN* (Physician Insurance Benefits per Capita)			
D.1......	.735	1.442^b (9.47)				
D.2......	.812	0.761^b (3.39)	0.254^b (3.70)			
D.3......	.819	1.465^b (10.89)		-1.576^b (-5.04)	-0.739^b (-4.26)	
D.4......	.754	1.270^b (3.62)			-0.259 (-0.93)	0.761 (1.43)
D.5......	.814	1.605^b (6.66)		-1.691^b (-5.04)	-0.838^b (-3.87)	-0.277 (-0.68)
D.6......	.823	1.060^b (3.28)	0.130 (1.48)	-1.116^a (-2.22)	-0.430 (-1.42)	
D.7......	.820	0.513 (0.77)	0.201 (1.82)	-0.596 (-0.82)	-0.030 (-0.06)	0.634 (0.91)

Note: Adjusted t statistics appear in parentheses.

[a] Significant at .05 level.   [b] Significant at .01 level.   [c] Linear variable.

Part A: Demand (Q*)

Income. Estimates of the income elasticity of demand vary over a wide range (0.04 to 0.57), but, taken together, the equations support the findings of previous investigators that physicians' services are considered to be very much of a necessity, with an income elasticity substantially below 1.0. Our results correspond particularly closely with those of Andersen and Benham [4], even though the units of observation are quite different (1966 state averages in one instance, 1964 family units in the other).[19] Simple regressions with income as the sole independent variable produce elasticities of 0.41 and 0.31, respectively, both coefficients significant at the 0.01 level. The results for multiple regressions are also similar. In our more successful demand equations (A.6-A.11) we observe considerably lower and much less significant income coefficients (0.20 in A.6, 0.04 in A.7), when indeed income appears at all. Andersen and Benham report a statistically insignificant income elasticity of 0.01 in multiple regression.[20]

It should, of course, be stressed that all of these values refer to the responsiveness of quantity—not of expenditures—to changes in income. The difference between the two is not trivial, given the tendency of AP to rise with income. A simple regression with per capita expenditures as the dependent variable yields an income coefficient of 0.96.

One factor that might possibly contribute to the very low income elasticity of demand is the high correlation of income with earnings, which, in turn, is a good indication of the price of time. Physicians' services are usually time-intensive, and this means that they are more costly to those with high earnings. Had we estimated the effect of income with earnings held constant, it is likely that a higher elasticity would result.[21] Unfortunately, the requisite state data are not available.

Chart 4

Ratio of Number of Physician Visits by Persons with Family Income Greater than $10,000 to Visits by Persons with Family Income Less than $3,000, by Age and Sex, 1966-67

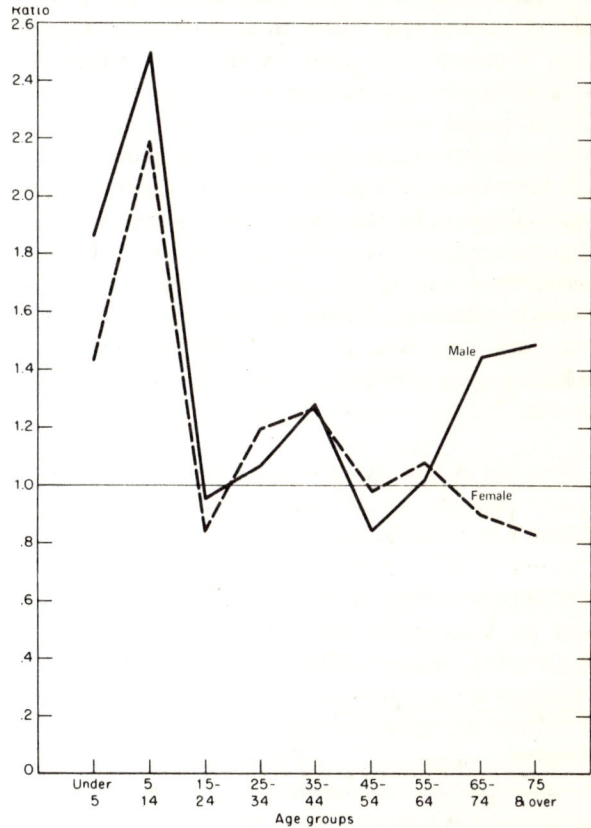

Source: U.S. Department of Health, Education, and Welfare, "Volume of Physician Visits, United States, July 1966-June 1967," *Vital and Health Statistics*, Series 10, No. 49, November 1968, p. 19.

The importance of the earnings factor can be appreciated from Chart 4, which shows, for various age and sex classes, the 1966 ratio of per capita physician visits made by persons with family incomes over $10,000 to those made by persons with family incomes under $3,000.

---

[19] Andersen and Benham, in their calculations for physician use, employ an estimate of "permanent income" as the independent variable rather than measured income, but this does not imply incomparability with our results since the transitory component of income is largely eliminated by using grouped data.

[20] Other demand elasticities reported in the literature are 0.62 and 0.21, respectively, in Feldstein [17] and Fein [15]. The elasticity implicit in Fein's book was computed by Herbert Klarman [27].

[21] Morris Silver postulates a *positive* relationship between earnings and *expenditures* for physicians' services, and his results bear this out [40]. But such a finding can be readily explained by the close association between earnings and price. It does not necessarily contradict our view that high earnings have a negative impact on the quantity component of expenditures.

Both sexes under the age of fourteen display very high visit-relatives; the same holds true for males aged sixty-five and over. In essence, earnings are held nearly constant (at approximately zero) as family income rises for these groups, allowing us to observe the effect on demand of income alone. The implicit income elasticities of demand are still less than 1.0, but hardly negligible. By contrast, income exerts no systematic influence upon visits of persons aged fifteen to sixty-four; the positive effect of income on demand, we believe, is nullified by the negative effect of earnings (i.e., the price of time). Also in accord with our expectations is the fact that among the twenty-five to sixty-four age group, where male labor-force participation rates are roughly twice as large as those for females, income exerts somewhat more of an influence on visits by females than visits by males. Indeed, only two of the eighteen age-sex categories behave in a contrary fashion to what we would expect under our hypothesis if it were the sole means of explaining age-sex differences in the effect of income on demand.[22]

Omission of quality differences from our quantity measure may also be exerting a downward bias on the estimated income elasticity, but the nature of medical education in this country (all recognized schools must have AMA accreditation, and National Board Examinations are increasingly employed as a state licensure requirement) makes it unlikely that state-to-state quality differences among physicians are an important factor. On balance, we believe that variations in earnings, on the one hand, and patients' *belief* in the essential nature of physicians' services, on the other, are responsible for the low income elasticity of demand.[23]

We should emphasize that problems of multicollinearity prevent any firm conclusions regarding the exact magnitude of the income coefficient. Thus, our income elasticities are consistently larger and generally more significant in the equations that do not consider MD* as a variable than in those that do. The great improvement in explanatory power which results with the introduction of MD* (A.6 versus A.2, A.7 versus A.5) and the

consistently high *t* statistic attaching to the physician variable lend credence to the latter specification. It is clear that, of the two variables, MD* is dominant, with income playing a comparatively minor role. These qualifications notwithstanding, there is nothing in these equations—regardless of what combination of variables we consider—to suggest an income elasticity even approaching 1.0. All of the evidence indicates that the demand for physicians' services is quite income-inelastic, though precisely to what degree we cannot accurately say.

Price and Insurance. The price elasticity of demand for physicians' services appears to be unusually low. None of the equations reported in Table 18.A show AP or NP coefficients exceeding (in absolute value) −0.36. The *t* statistics on the price variables indicate that a high degree of confidence can be placed in this finding. Our result parallels Paul Feldstein's finding [17] of a low demand price elasticity of −0.19, also significantly different from zero.[24]

There are three principal explanations for the relative insensitivity of demand to changes in price. First, it should be remembered that the demand for physicians' services is derived from the consumer's demand for health. Michael Grossman has estimated the price elasticity of demand for health at −0.5 [22], which seems reasonable, given the absence of any close substitutes for health. The price elasticity of demand for a derived input must be lower than for the final commodity unless there are important possibilities of substitution with other inputs. This leads to the second explanation, namely, that there are many legal and psychological barriers against the substitution of persons without the M.D. degree in the physicians's role, even though such persons might be good substitutes in a technical sense. Similarly, there are many factors other than medical manpower that contribute to the individual's production of health, including diet, housing, recreation, and education. These may, in fact, be excellent alternatives to physicians' services in the long run, but may not be so regarded by the patient.[25]

Finally, it should be noted that the price paid is only part of the total cost of physicians' services to the

---

[22] Visit-relatives for women sixty-five to seventy-five and seventy-five and over rise rapidly, as predicted, over low income classes, but then fall even more steeply, for some unknown reason, over high income classes.

[23] This is not to say that all, or even most, physicians' services are technically essential for health. To *believe* in their efficacy is sufficient to make the average individual treat them as a necessity in his budget.

---

[24] Feldstein's study pertained to physician visits by families in 1953.

[25] The same argument can be made with regard to "negative inputs" in the production of health, including such consumption items as tobacco, alcohol, narcotics, and (occasionally) motor vehicles.

patient. In addition to possible inconvenience, the patient must reckon with costs of transportation and, more important, time spent in travel, waiting, and during the visit itself. These indirect costs (IC) vary greatly from individual to individual, though in general we would expect a positive association between them and the direct cost of a visit (AP) because IC is closely dependent upon the price of time, AP varies with income, and both income and the price of time are highly correlated with earnings. In the event that IC and AP are perfectly correlated, variations in AP are exactly proportional to variations in the total price of a visit and the AP coefficients we estimate are not biased, despite the omission of an IC variable. If, however, IC tends to rise faster than AP, we are underestimating the true interstate variation in price and thereby overestimating the price elasticity of demand, and vice versa. The direction of possible bias from this source is not ascertainable.

The relevance of insurance to demand is tested in two ways. We first investigate the role of insurance using the BEN* variable. Unfortunately, strong multicollinearity between income and benefits prevents any conclusions on this score. The $\bar{R}^2$ is essentially unchanged, whether we employ income, benefits, or both in the demand regression (A.2-A.4); while either variable alone is highly significant, both show much lower t values when they appear jointly. It is impossible to infer how much of the observed variation in Q* is attributable to each of these variables, or what the true coefficients of each are.

NP is superior to BEN* as a measure of insurance because of its much smaller correlation with INC* (0.14 versus 0.86). Using NP we may consider all economic influences on demand simultaneously (i.e., income, average price, and insurance, the latter two embodied in the NP variable). With insurance thus accounted for, we observe a somewhat smaller but still very significant income elasticity as compared to the case of income and average price considered alone (A.5 versus A.2). The high correlation between AP and NP nonetheless complicates the critical judgment as to whether insurance per se is important to demand. In some instances AP is the stronger variable (A.6 versus A.5), while in others the situation is reversed and NP is stronger (A.8 versus A.9). But in any case, the price elasticity of demand is not much affected by the choice between these two price variables.

What we can say with assurance concerning the role of insurance in demand is that the elasticity of Q* with respect to BEN* is, at most, fairly low. That is, even under the extreme assumption that INC* is of *no* real importance in this relation, the elasticity with respect to BEN* is only 0.31. The very large t statistic on BEN* in A.4 indicates not only that this coefficient is significantly greater than 0, but also that it is significantly less than 0.4. Such a finding is not in line with our prior notions concerning the effect of insurance, despite the fact that in at least one instance comparable findings have been reported in the literature.[26] Some discussion of possible explanations is, therefore, in order.

First, the prevailing impression about insurance is that it induces higher utilization by lowering the price faced by the consumer. Yet if this is the mechanism through which insurance operates on demand, and if demand is price-inelastic, as we have found the case to be, it is to be expected that demand will also be insurance-inelastic. For example, if benefits initially reimburse 40 per cent of average price, a 1 per cent rise in BEN* will produce a 0.67 per cent fall in NP (from 0.60 AP to 0.596 AP). With a (net) price elasticity of −0.20, this will result in only a 0.13 per cent rise in Q* (close to the 0.18 rise shown by A.3). On the other hand, if demand were highly responsive to price changes, say with an elasticity of −1.5, the same 1 per cent rise in BEN* would call forth a 1.00 per cent rise in Q*. It should be noted that we would expect the effect of insurance on demand to be greater among persons with a very low or negligible price of time (the young, the elderly, the unemployed), because incremental insurance benefits for them result in a much larger percentage change in the full price of a visit.

A second factor is that private insurance for physicians' services is usually heavily biased toward coverage of relatively nondiscretionary care. Surgical procedures and in-hospital care are far more likely to be reimbursed than routine office visits or preventive services [34]; This restriction in coverage may greatly reduce the impact of insurance relative to what it might have been.

Physicians. The highly significant role of MD* in the demand equation requires some discussion. It cannot be attributed to a supply-induced fall in the

---

[26] Paul Feldstein [17] uses an insurance variable (the ratio of benefits to expenditures) in his demand analysis. Contrary to his expectations, the elasticity is negative, though insignificant. Regrettably, no discussion of this finding appears in the text.

physician's fee because price (AP or NP) is already held constant. Rather, it seems to be the result of the following forces.

First, an increase in MD* is likely to reduce the average distance separating patient and physician, as well as the average waiting time. The consequent saving in time and transportation expense lowers the total cost of a visit to the patient even if fees are held constant. Given a low price elasticity of demand, however, this factor alone is insufficient to account for the magnitude of the MD* coefficient.

A second possibility is that physicians themselves inflate demand whenever the supply of medical manpower is relatively slack. This thesis is put forth persuasively by Eli Ginzberg: ". . . the supply of medical resources has thus far effectively generated its own demand. . . . Much unnecessary surgery continues to be performed. . . . There is substantial overdoctoring for a host of diseases, including, in particular, infections of the upper respiratory tract. . . . [physicians] usually have wide margins of discretion about whether to recommend that a patient return to the office for one or more follow-up visits [21]."

A supply-induced demand change is fully sufficient as an explanation for the role of MD* in the Q* equations of Table 18.A; if verified, its implications for policy are profound. Evidence that the additional physicians' services provided under loose supply conditions are, in fact, of a marginal nature is presented in the discussion of the effect of physicians' services on health in section 2.6. This much is to be expected if, as Ginzberg also suggests, physicians gravitate towards the more serious cases as their supply becomes taut.

A third possible explanation for the importance of MD* is the existence of permanent excess demand for physicians' services. This is the thesis advanced by Martin Feldstein [16], whose time series analysis of this market yielded positive demand price elasticities (as high as 1.67), inconsistent with an equilibrium hypothesis. Feldstein's negative and significant insurance elasticities and his occasionally negative income elasticities are likewise inexplicable under normal market conditions. In our view, a much simpler interpretation of Feldstein's results is the failure to take account of technological change, which shifted the demand curve to the right over time, and not at a constant rate. Since the cross-section regressions, which essentially hold technology constant,

are readily interpretable under the assumption of market equilibrium, we see no reason to substitute either here or in the time series the less defensible explanation of permanent excess demand.

Hospital Bed Supply. Introducing BEDS* into any of the demand equations discussed above seriously affects the conclusions to be drawn regarding price (either AP or NP). A.10 is illustrative: The price coefficient approaches zero (in some equations it actually becomes positive) and the variable loses all statistical significance. Indeed, the "best" demand equations, in terms of sheer explanatory power ($\overline{R}^2$), is one in which price, income, and insurance have all been dropped and only MD* and BEDS* appear (A.11).

Accepting the results of A.11 on face value may nonetheless be seriously misleading. To be sure, a rationale is advanced here in support of a causal relationship running from bed supply to demand for physicians' services. That is, the services of hospitals and of physicians are in many ways a joint consumption item, and thus an increase in the former serving to meet a backlog in *its* demand will permit an expanded consumption of physicians' services, desired but technically unfeasible previously due to the unavailability of the requisite hospital facilities. Beyond this, if the frequent allegation is true that the supply of hospital beds tends to create its own demand, it follows that any increase in BEDS*, even if wholly unrelated to the prevailing demand for hospitalization, will (indirectly) raise Q* as well.

The trouble with this explanation for the role of BEDS* in the Q* equation is that it takes no account of the fact that the relationship between these two variables is inherently biased by the very method used to construct Q*. Hospital days per capita comprise one of the three components of the quantity series, and because there is so little interstate variation in occupancy rates, days are almost entirely proportional to bed capacity. In our judgment, BEDS* is probably significant in the Q* equation not so much because it bears a causal relationship to the dependent variable but rather because of the statistical dependence of Q* upon BEDS*. Equations in section A that do not include BEDS* are probably more accurate indications of the true determinants of demand for this reason.

Part B: Supply of Physicians (MD*)

Medical schools, price, hospital bed supply, and per capita income are the principal factors influencing physicians' locational decisions (Table 18.B). Collinearity among the last three of these variables makes it difficult to determine precisely the specific effect of each, but the four together account for about 78 per cent of the variation in MD*.

The role of the medical school in physician location is twofold. As a center of education it draws doctors-to-be to the state, and its affiliated hospitals attract interns and residents. Professional contacts are established, and young families take root. As a major medical center, it generally promises superior staff and facilities in its teaching hospitals. Regardless of where they trained, physicians may find it advantageous to have such a complex within close proximity of their practice, for it allows them to arrange referrals and consultations while maintaining contact with the patient. Our estimated coefficient, highly significant in all but two cases, indicates that on the average one additional medical school in a state raises the number of physicians practicing there by about 4 per cent.

A glance at equations B.2-B.8 makes apparent the presence of collinearity among the three other important location variables. Price is highly significant, with coefficients ranging from 0.83 to 1.14, in those equations where it appears alone with MED SCLS or where BEDS* is also present (B.3, B.6, B.7), but with BEDS* dropped and INC* retained, the price coefficient falls considerably and loses its significance (B.5). In like fashion, INC* is a significant variable, with an elasticity of 0.49 to 0.76, when it appears alone with MED SCLS or in conjunction with either AP or BEDS* (B.2, B.5, B.8), but both its coefficient and its adjusted t statistic plummet when all four variables enter the equation (B.6). Similarly, BEDS* is significant if, and only if, AP also appears in the equation (B.6 and B.7, but not B.4 or B.8). It is with caution, therefore, that we proceed to a discussion of these results.

Our average price measure is clearly superior as a supply variable in this context to physician gross income, the monetary incentive variable employed by Benham, Maurizi, and Reder [7]. In their analysis the two-stage least squares method was utilized to estimate demand and supply equations for the number of

physicians in each state in 1950, but, while physician income had a positive sign in the supply equation, it was not statistically significant. This is as expected: business receipts are positively related to workload as well as to price, and it is surely unreasonable to expect doctors to be attracted to states where they can anticipate little leisure time. If anything, the opposite hypothesis merits consideration, and we investigate this possibility. Unlike the demand equations, where there was some question regarding the specification of the relevent price variable itself (AP or NP), AP is obviously the correct choice in this case, since it matters little, if at all, to the supplier of services who is paying the bills he sends out.

INC* serves in the physician supply equation as a general taste variable rather than as an indication of financial inducements to settlement, since price is also held constant. As predicted, the life style available in high-income states does appear to exercise some influence over the location of physicians.[27] Hospital bed supply—which is probably a proxy in a more general sense for the whole range of medical facilities and auxiliary personnel—also appears to be an important nonpecuniary consideration in physicians' location decisions.

No support is found for the view that physicians actually shun states where the average physician workload is high. The endogenous $\hat{Q}/MD$ variable bears the anticipated negative sign but never approaches significance, and its inclusion, in fact, only serves to reduce the adjusted R^2 of the regression (B.9 versus B.7, B.10 versus B.6). That certain areas, both rural and urban

---

[27] Because the total number of practicing physicians in the country (MD_t) is constant in cross-section, an analysis such as this can only throw light on the reasons for geographic variation in this total. Given the presence of substantial barriers to entry into medicine, it is wholly unwarranted to conclude that the same behavioral patterns observed for physicians in cross-section will also apply over time in the determination of MD_t. In all probability, a proportional change in INC* across all states would have no effect on MD_t or on the particular state levels of $MD*_{it}$. It follows that only variations in *relative* income are potentially influential in determining the geographic distribution of a given number of physicians. The relative attractiveness of a state is best represented by $\frac{INC_i^*}{\overline{INC^*}}$, where the denominator represents mean per capita income for the sample. Replacing our INC* variables with this relative income measure would have no effect on the estimated elasticities because the corresponding values of both variables are proportional in any one year. But it is best kept in mind that the INC* variable of Table 18.B should only be interpreted in a relative sense.

ghetto, are unpopular with physicians is indisputable, but fear of overwork does not appear to be a factor in their judgment.

Part C: Quantity per Physician (Q/MD)

The number of physicians per capita is the only variable tested that clearly has a significant impact on physician productivity. It alone accounts for 60 per cent of the variation in Q/MD. The coefficient of the MD* variable indicates that about two-thirds of the incremental supply of physicians' services that might be expected to ensue with an increase in the number of physicians practicing in a state will be effectively nullified by a reduction in output of the average practitioner. These results suggest that increases in the number of physicians in a state, whether resulting from shifts in distribution or expansion of the total stock, may actually result in *higher* prices for physicians' services. According to the regressions, a 10 per cent rise in MD* will lead to a 4 per cent rise in demand as the new physicians create a market for their services, but the supply of services may rise by as little as 3 1/3 per cent once resident doctors have adjusted to the decreased urgency of unattended cases and opted for a reduction in their activity.

The price elasticity of supply per physician is probably low. Only a very small degree of confidence can attach to the initial finding of a negative price elasticity. Some collinearity between AP and MD* is present, as demonstrated by the reduced *t* statistic of each when they appear jointly (C.1 and C.2 versus C.3); although C.3, with price included, is superior to C.2, C.4 is inferior to C.5. These results are not unlike those reported by Martin Feldstein [16]: price coefficients in his supply-per-physician equations range from −0.28 to −1.91, with only the higher (absolute) values achieving significance at the 5 per cent level. In any case, we find no support for the hypothesis that higher prices induce *additional* services from physicians already located in a state.

Adding BEDS* to the productivity equation with only MD* in it increases the explanatory power by a fair amount (C.5 versus C.2), but the BEDS* coefficient is statistically insignificant and of a low magnitude.

Part D: Insurance (BEN*)

The purchase of physician insurance by consumers, as distinct from physician care itself, appears to be very sensitive to variations in personal income. We find elasticities ranging from 0.76 to 1.61, and in all cases but one they are significant at the 1 per cent level (the exception is D.7, where the simultaneous presence of so many independent variables cancels the significance of each and also lowers the INC* elasticity).

Three other hypotheses are investigated relating to the determinants of BEN*. Again, because of high correlations among the independent variables, we test these theories one at a time before assessing their effects in combination.

The degree of unionization has a small but important effect on BEN*, raising the $\bar{R}^2$ from 0.74 in D.1 to 0.81 in D.2. This conclusion is weakened when PRM/BEN and AP also appear in the equation, but even then the $\bar{R}^2$ is improved by inclusion of UNION* (D.6 versus D.3).

The purchase of insurance seems to be very responsive to its price, PIV. This composite variable is dependent both upon the average price of physicians' services and upon the cost of one dollar of insurance benefits. As predicted by this hypothesis, the coefficients of AP and PRM/BEN are each negative and highly significant in D.3. Deducting 1.0 from the estimated AP coefficient allows us to interpret the equation as a representation of the demand for insured visit equivalents (i.e., BEN*/AP). We see that the price elasticity of demand, as indicated by both PIV components, appears to be quite high, on the order of −1.58 to −1.74.[28] Apparently, the decision to purchase medical insurance is influenced much more by income and price than is the decision to purchase physicians' services.

We find no support for the financial-protection theory of insurance, which holds that the amount of insurance people wish to carry varies directly with the level of anticipated expenditures they are insuring against. This theory predicts equal, positive coefficients of approximately 1.0 for both AP and Q*,[29] yet we find

---

[28] Because of some collinearity between these variables and UNION*, the significance level of each of the three is diminished in D.6, and the coefficients somewhat lower as well.

[29] It may be argued that insurance purchases are sensitive both to their price and to anticipated expenditures levels, and that AP therefore serves in a dual capacity in the BEN* regression. If this is correct, the AP coefficient we observe should be on the order of -0.6(+1.0 for the expenditures theory and -1.6 for the price theory). This possibility is tested and rejected in D.5, for the PRM/BEN and AP coefficients are essentially unchanged from their values in D.3, while Q* is now negative.

in D.4 that the coefficient of AP is negative, while that of Q* is positive but not statistically significant. Dropping Q* from the regression brings about a slight improvement in the $\overline{R}^2$ (D.7 versus D.6, D.5 versus D.3) and permits a much less ambiguous interpretation of the role of AP in insurance purchases. It is only because of its dependence upon AP that insurance is endogenous to this system.

Because of the many ambiguities complicating the interpretation of most of these regression equations, we feel it wisest to refrain from presenting a reduced-form version of the model.[30] We have seen that two of the exogenous variables—BEDS* and INC*—lend themselves to more than one interpretation, depending upon the equation in which they appear, but such distinctions would be lost in a reduced form. More serious is the problem of multicollinearity. The consequent instability of coefficient estimates is troublesome enough in the interpretation of individual regression equations, but then at least it is known which variables must be approached with caution. In a reduced form, because of the intricate pattern of substitutions, this instability may be magnified manyfold and its repercussions felt throughout the entire system. Depending upon the choice of equations to represent the model, numerous versions of the reduced form are possible, some with sharply contrasting implications. Under the circumstances, it seems preferable to state the limitations of our knowledge rather than compound the possibility of error.

2.6 The Effect on Health

The degree to which variations in the quantity of physicians' services consumed affect health status, i.e., Health = f(Q*, . . .), is a matter of prime concern. A priori considerations suggest that causality might run in the reverse direction as well, from health to demand [Q* = g(Health, . . .)]. If so, two-stage least squares would be the recommended method for determining the effect of quantity on health, with the predicted value of the endogenous Q* variable entering the health regressions and vice versa. In the preliminary large-scale model described in 2.2, this procedure was adopted. As noted earlier, however, tests based upon this model lent no support to the hypothesis that variations in health

contribute to interstate variations in the demand for physicians' services. Hence, coefficients obtained from ordinary least squares regressions of health on Q* should not be biased.[31]

Two dependent variables have been chosen to represent health status in these regressions: the crude death rate (DTH RT) and the infant mortality rate (INF MRT). The independent variables include factors of a general nature—income, education, per cent black, and per cent aged (this last only in the DTH RT equations)—and factors specifically related to the consumption of physicians' services. In addition to Q*, we test MD* and per capita expenditures for physicians' services (EXP*) in this equation. The first of these is, theoretically, the desired variable, but because of possible measurement errors we do not rely upon it exclusively. No two of these physician variables rely upon the same data base.

The most important conclusion we can draw from the regressions of Table 19 is that, other things being equal, variation in the consumption of physicians' services does not seem to have any significant effect on health, as measured by either the crude death rate or the infant mortality rate. This finding is consistent with the work of previous investigators concerning the relative unimportance of medical care (not restricted to physicians' services) as a determinant of interstate variations in death rates [5].

Higher educational levels are very strongly associated with lower crude death rates. Education is also negatively related to infant mortality, but not statistically significant.[32] Contrary to what many would expect, per capita income is positively related to the crude death rate after controlling for the effect of education. It is, however, negatively related to infant mortality. These results for education and income confirm the findings of

---

[30] In a reduced form, individual regression equations are solved so that Q* and AP can be expressed wholly in terms of the exogenous variables.

[31] Two-stage regressions with health as the dependent variable are not feasible within the context of the present model. This is because the exogenous determinants of health do not appear in the model. Their exclusion was based upon the insignificance of health itself in the demand equation. To reintroduce health would necessitate bringing back into the model several exogenous variables that bear no demonstrable relationship to the market for physicians' services, and, as explained in 2.2, this, in turn, would impart a bias to all of the first-stage predicted endogenous variables.

[32] Our analysis implicitly assumes causality to run only from education to health, but this is not necessarily the case. See the forthcoming paper by Victor Fuchs and Michael Grossman [20].

TABLE 19

Results of Weighted, Logarithmic Health Regressions, Ordinary Least Squares, Interstate Model, 1966 (N=33)

(*t* values in parentheses)

Equation		$\bar{R}^2$	%AGED[a]	INC*	%BLK[a]	EDUC	Q*	MD*	EXP*
Part A									
DTH RT	DR. 1	.560	0.055[b] (6.41)	-0.008 (-0.12)					
	DR. 2	.679	0.061[b] (8.25)			-0.364[b] (-3.33)			
	DR. 3	.814	0.060[b] (10.71)	0.333[b] (4.79)		-0.823[b] (-6.49)			
	DR. 4	.811	0.062[b] (9.90)	0.354[b] (4.68)	0.001 (0.73)	-0.780[b] (-5.54)			
	DR. 5	.804	0.062[b] (9.31)	0.347[b] (3.67)	0.001 (0.71)	-0.779[b] (-5.42)	0.016 (0.13)		
	DR. 6	.811	0.062[b] (9.93)	0.404[b] (4.44)	0.001 (0.87)	-0.739[b] (-5.04)		-0.057 (-0.99)	
	DR. 7	.815	0.059[b] (8.95)	0.391[b] (4.85)	0.001 (0.88)	-0.658[b] (-3.86)			-0.079 (-1.24)
Part B									
INF MRT	IM. 1	.796		-0.144 (-1.68)	0.011[b] (6.47)				
	IM. 2	.787			0.011[b] (6.33)	-0.196 (-1.19)			
	IM. 3	.791		-0.122 (-1.22)	0.010[b] (5.55)	-0.083 (-0.44)			
	IM. 4	.785		-0.089 (-0.73)	0.010[b] (5.43)	-0.090 (-0.47)	-0.079 (-0.50)		
	IM. 5	.783		-0.132 (-1.08)	0.010[b] (5.38)	-0.090 (-0.46)		0.011 (0.14)	
	IM. 6	.787		-0.152 (-1.38)	0.010[b] (5.10)	-0.172 (-0.75)			0.056 (0.69)

[a] Linear variable.
[b] Significant at .01 level.

Fuchs [19], Grossman [22], and Auster, Leveson, and Sarachek [5]. The per cent black is positively associated with both death variables, but the effect is much greater with respect to infant mortality.

2.7 Conclusion

In Part 2 we have presented a formal econometric model of the market for physicians' services in 1966, using cross-sectional data for our estimates. The findings, which must be regarded as tentative because of the limited quantity and uneven quality of available data, tend to be consistent with, and give support to, the inferences drawn from the time series examined in Part 1.

The demand for physicians' services appears to be significantly influenced by the number of physicians available. The effect exerted on demand by supply appears to be stronger than that of income, price, or insurance coverage. Physician supply, across states, is positively related to price, the presence of medical schools and hospital beds, and the educational, cultural, and recreational milieu. The quantity of service produced per physician is negatively related to the number of physicians in an area. It does not increase in response to higher fees. The demand for medical insurance, unlike the demand for physicians' services, does appear to be quite sensitive to differences in income. It is also significantly related to the price of insurance and to unionization. Finally, interstate differences in infant mortality and overall death rates are not significantly related to the number of physicians, to the quantity of their services, or to expenditures.

If subsequent research should confirm these findings, the implications for public policy are substantial. According to a widespread view, large increases in the number of physicians will drive down the price of, and expenditures for, physicians' services, will diminish the inequality in their location, provide a proportionate increase in the quantity of services, and make a substantial contribution to improved health levels. The model and data we have examined do not provide any support for this view.

Appendix A. Time Series: Sources and Methods

Expenditures: Data on national expenditures for physicians' services are published periodically by the Social Security Administration in the *Social Security Bulletin* and in *Research and Statistics Note.* See, for example, [11] and [8]. The series used in this paper (Table 1) represents the most recent official revision of these figures [12].

The principal component of this expenditures series is gross business receipts of physicians in private practice (sole proprietorships, partnerships, and corporations) reported to the Internal Revenue Service. Also included are the estimated gross receipts of osteopaths, a share of the gross of medical and dental laboratories (estimated to represent patient payments to them), and estimated expenses of group-practice prepayment plans in providing physicians' services (to the extent that these are not included in physicians' gross self-employment income). Estimated receipts of physicians for making life insurance examinations are deducted from the above. It should be noted that the expenditures series so obtained does not represent the market value of the services of *all* practicing physicians. Excluded are the salaries of public and private hospital staff physicians (considered a component of hospital care); salaries of physicians in public health departments (classed with government public health expenditures); and salaries of physicians in the Armed Forces and Indian Health Service (classed as expenditures for "medical activities in Federal units other than hospitals") [35].

Public expenditures: Federal, state, and local payments for the services of private practice physicians. These data are published regularly by the Social Security Administration, along with the data on total expenditures. We have used the most recent revision of these figures [12].

Customary price: Average annual level of the index of physicians' fees of the Consumer Price Index [60].

Average price: See Appendix B.

Insurance: Private health insurance benefit payments for surgical and regular medical expenses (including major medical payments for these purposes). Annual data are published by the Health Insurance Institute [23]. For 1952-60, see [23, 1961 edition, p. 41]; for 1960-68, see [23, 1969 edition, p. 35]. For 1948-51, data published in [23] only apply to commercial insurance companies and Blue Shield—they do not include benefits paid by Blue Cross or by independent hospital-medical plans. We therefore estimate a total for these years by assuming that the ratio of Blue Shield benefits to payments made by all noncommercial insurers was the same in 1948-51 as in the average of the two succeeding years (71.4 per cent in 1952, 71.8 per cent in 1953). This gives us an estimate of benefits paid by noncommercial sources. Adding this to the benefit figure for insurance companies, we have total private insurance benefits for physicians' services for these four years.

Third-party payments: The sum of public expenditures and private insurance benefits.

Net price: The sum payable by the patient himself for one standard visit. Net price is computed as average price multiplied by the ratio of direct expenditures (total expenditures less third-party payments) to total expenditures.

Persons insured: The number of individuals with at least one form of private insurance coverage for physician expenses. This is estimated as the number of persons covered by surgical insurance policies plus 2 per cent of those with regular medical policies plus 2 per cent of those with major medical policies [23]. An explanation of this formula is included in Appendix B, under variable I_t.

Quantity: Expenditures divided by the average price index.

Population series: U.S. civilian resident population, July 1 of each year. Alaska and Hawaii are included beginning 1959. For 1948-58, see [46]; for 1959-67, see [47]; and for 1968, see [45].

Real disposable personal income: [14].

Demographic index—visits: For 1948, 1956, 1966, and 1968, the percentage of the total population in each of twelve age-sex classes [47: 1949, 1957, 1967, and 1969 editions] was weighted by average per capita physician visits for that class, July 1963-June 1964 [56, Table 7], to arrive at a predicted per capita visit figure for each year.

Demographic Index—expenditures: For 1948, 1956, 1966, and 1968, the percentage of the total population in each of twelve age-sex classes was weighted by average per capita expenditures for physicians' services for that class, 1962 [55, Table 1], to arrive at a predicted per capita expenditures figure for each year.

Real gross national product (GNP): GNP [14, p. 177] divided by GNP implicit price deflator [14, p. 180].

Persons engaged (total economy): For 1948-65, [48, pp. 112-13]; for 1966-68, [50].

Crude death rate: A three-year average, centered on the given year, of the number of deaths per 1,000 population. For 1949-67, see [47]; for 1968, see [32].

Crude death rate, cancer and heart disease: A three-year moving average. For 1949-67, see [47].

Average length of stay (days): For nonfederal, short-term general hospitals and other special hospitals [25, various issues].

Hospital days: Product of admissions and average length of stay, for nonfederal, short-term general hospitals and other special hospitals [25, various issues].

Physicians: The basic series used in the computation of expenditures per physician and of quantity per physician (Tables 7 and 9) refers to physicians in private practice. Prior to 1959 the figures apply to the forty-eight states and the District of Columbia; beginning with that year the data are for fifty states and the District of Columbia. The sources for this series, as well as for the complete categorization of all U.S. physicians by activity, are [31, p. 3] for 1949, 1955, 1957, and 1959, and [2] for 1963, 1966, and 1967.

Specialists: Private practice physicians who are full-time specialists [31], [2]. Prior to 1963 the number of private practice physicians with a part-time specialty was steadily shrinking relative to the number with full-time specialty. Since then the AMA statistics only distinguish "specialists" and general practitioners, with no explanation given as to the current classification of those physicians who formerly would have fallen into the part-time specialist category.

General practitioners: [31], [2]. Prior to 1963 the figure includes part-time specialists.

Per cent partners: Number of physicians filing partnership returns as a per cent of all physicians filing business income tax returns for medical practice [33, p. 74].

Visits per physician: Applies to self-employed physicians under sixty-five years of age. In 1947, the average physician had 25.1 visits per day and worked 6 days a week, 48.75 weeks per year, giving a total of 7,342 visits per year. By 1968, the median number of visits per week had fallen to 131 and the median number of weeks worked to 47.9 (1967), for a total of 6,275 visits per year. [29, issues of February 1948, March 1948, May 1949, April 1, 1968, and December 8, 1969].

Quantity per visit: The increase in the quantity of physicians' services per visit which has occurred over time can be decomposed into an increase in quantity attributable to the shift toward specialization—analogous to an increase in quality insofar as specialists are higher-quality physicians—and a residual representing the pure productivity increase for physicians of a given level of training. The quality of the average visit in a given year is computed by determining the per cent of total visits performed by each kind of practitioner, and then weighting specialists' visits according to their higher average receipts, in this case 1.93 (see Appendix C, variable a). Thus

$$QL = \frac{V_g G + a V_s S}{V_g G + V_s S}$$

where QL = quality of the average visit; V_g, V_s = visits per G. P., visits per specialist; G, S = number of G. P.'s, number of specialists; a = "quality" of a specialist's visit relative to one by a G. P. (measured by ratio of average gross receipts per visit). In 1947, G. P.'s (67.7 per cent of the total) made 27 visits per day, while specialists made only 22 [29, May 1949]; in 1966, G. P.'s (34.2 per cent of total) were making 154 visits per week, specialists, 91 per week [29, Feb. 6, 1967]. These data cover solo practitioners only. Thus, the average quality of a visit rose from 1.26 to 1.49 over this nineteen-year period (a rate of 0.9 per cent per year) as a result of the shift to specialization.

Average business expenses per physician: Average gross business receipts per physician minus average net profit per physician, as reported to the Internal Revenue Service [33, p. 75].

Expenditures for dental services: [28].

Fee index for dental services: [28].

Dentists: [33].

Table A-1

Public Expenditures and Insurance, 1948-68

Year	Public Expenditures for Physicians' Services (Millions of $)	Private Medical Insurance Benefits (Millions of $)	Persons with Private Medical Insurance Coverage (Millions)
1948	$116	$158	34.3
1949	126	196	41.5
1950	143	294	54.6
1951	164	413	65.4
1952	184	537	73.2
1953	207	655	81.9
1954	230	735	86.9
1955	248	840	90.1
1956	272	955	99.5
1957	310	1,178	106.9
1958	348	1,315	109.4
1959	371	1,474	114.9
1960	366	1,642	119.6
1961	407	1,878	125.5
1962	446	2,084	129.6
1963	475	2,311	134.8
1964	511	2,577	138.5
1965	552	2,876	143.8
1966	785	3,086	148.2
1967	1,989	3,535	154.1
1968	2,638	3,761	159.6

Table A-2

Physicians, by Type of Practice, 1947-68

Year	Physicians in Private Practice	Specialists in Private Practice	Per Cent in Partnership Practice	Average Business Expenses per Physician
1947	148,627[a]	47,943	5.8	$6,443
1948	149,519[a]	51,300[a]		
1949	150,417	54,891		
1950				
1951				
1952				
1953			9.5	8,755
1954				
1955	152,305	67,114		
1956	153,825[a]		14.0[b]	
1957	155,827	74,384	12.1[b]	11,113
1958			15.5[b]	12,139
1959	160,592	78,635	12.6	12,707
1960	164,847[a]		16.8	12,768
1961			16.0[b]	13,038
1962			15.1	13,405
1963	178,295	110,204	16.3	14,379
1964			22.4	15,794
1965			22.2	16,480
1966	185,847	122,270	22.7	17,450
1967	188,772	126,508		
1968	191,037[a]			

[a] Interpolated or extrapolated.
[b] Estimated by Louis S. Reed, [33].

Appendix B. Time Series: Derivation of Average Price

Since we have neither time series data on the average price actually received per visit nor the means to obtain such a series in dollar terms,[1] an indirect approach must be adopted in the construction of an average price index. The method followed here consists of estimating the ratio of AP to CP in each year and then multiplying this by the known CP index to obtain an index of average price.

By definition, AP_t/CP_t equals the ratio of expenditures for physicians services to the total *value* of those services, valuing services at their customary price. By assumption, this ratio is entirely dependent upon the extent of insurance coverage in the population, and must equal 1 if all services are fully reimbursed. Thus

$$\frac{AP_t}{CP_t} = \frac{U_{It}\,I_t\,K_t\,CP_t + U_{Nt}\,N_t\,k\,CP_t}{U_{It}\,I_t\,CP_t + U_{Nt}\,N_t\,CP_t}$$

$$= \frac{U_t\,I_t\,K_t + N_t\,k}{U_t\,I_t + N_t} \qquad (1)$$

where U_{It}, U_{Nt} = utilization of services per insured, and per uninsured, in year t;

U_t = U_{It}/U_{Nt}, the utilization ratio;

I_t, N_t = number of insured, and of uninsured, persons in year t;

K_t = fraction of CP paid by insured persons, year t; and

k = fraction of CP paid by uninsured persons (assumed constant).

The basic formula for computation of an AP index was first proposed by Martin Feldstein [16], and we owe much to his work in this area. However, in the assumptions and methods used to develop the requisite series our approach differs from his in several important respects. In particular:

---

[1] Dividing expenditures by the total number of visits, adjusted for variations in the nature of the average visit, is the method used to obtain price in the cross section and theoretically would be equally applicable for the time series as well. Unfortunately, data regarding the total number of physician visits are available for very few years in the period under consideration, and these come from several different sources (some sampling physicians, others sampling patients).

1. Feldstein assumes U_t to be constant over time, unaffected by the extent to which insured persons are reimbursed for their expenditures. We assume, rather, that the relative utilization of insured persons is directly proportional to the real amount of insurance benefits they receive.

2. Since U_t is derived by comparing actual utilization patterns of insured and uninsured persons (in Feldstein's paper as well as in ours), the appropriate I_t series should be the number of persons with any private insurance coverage for physician expenses. Feldstein, however, employs a weighted average of the number of persons covered under the three different kinds of policies, surgical (S), regular medical (RM), and major medical (MM), using as weights the benefits paid under each kind of policy. Consequently, his measure of I_t is necessarily understated, and the degree of understatement may vary from year to year.

3. Feldstein assumes that insured persons pay the full customary price for all services received, regardless of whether or not a particular service is covered under their insurance policy (i.e., $K_t = 1$, every year). We, on the other hand, assume insured persons to have a payment ratio of 1 only to the extent that the services they purchase are reimbursed; on uninsured services we assume their payments ratio to be less than 1, though greater than that of uninsured persons.

What follows below is a detailed discussion of the manner in which each of the component series of equation (1) is constructed.

I_t: Ideally, we would like I_t to be the per cent of the population with any physician expense protection. Unfortunately, the published statistics [23] do not include annual data on the extent of duplication among persons covered under the three kinds of policies. To estimate this duplication, we consider the findings of two nationwide surveys of health services conducted in 1963, one by the Health Information Foundation and National Opinion Research Center [3], the other by the National Health Survey of the U.S. Public Health Service [54]. We know from [3] that 66 per cent of the population has S and/or RM coverage, and from [23] and [3] that 65 per cent had S. Since 55 per cent of the population had RM in that year [54], only about 2 per cent of persons with RM (1/55) were not also covered by S.

We know further from [3] that 22 per cent of the population had MM coverage, while only 69 per cent of the population had health insurance of any kind, including hospital expense protection. Thus, a maximum of 3 per cent (69-66) of the population had MM as their sole form of physician expense coverage. However, it is most unreasonable to assume the minimum amount of overlap possible between the MM and S-RM categories, particularly since the former is generally regarded as supplementary to other forms of health insurance. Most likely, fewer than ½ per cent of the population, or about 2 per cent of those with MM, had MM but *not* S or RM. Thus, we estimate an annual I_t series by summing the number of persons with S + 2 per cent of the number with RM + 2 per cent of the number with MM.

Government insurance programs should have the same impact on *AP/CP* as private insurance. Prior to the institution of Medicare and Medicaid in 1966, however, public expenditures for physicians' services were relatively small in amount and widely dispersed through the population by a multiplicity of programs; there are no figures on the number of persons affected by one or more of these programs.[2] Since 1966 most public expenditures for physicians' services have been directed towards two well-defined population groups, the elderly and the medically indigent. We have expanded our I_t figure for these years to include the number of persons covered by Medicare Part B (physician insurance) but *not* also covered by private insurance, in keeping with the concept of I_t defined above (persons covered under *any* policy). Annual data on private insurance coverage of the elderly, by type of policy, are from [23]. Statistics on enrollment in Medicare Part B are from [36]; we assume that all elderly persons with private coverage have Medicare as well. Unfortunately, it has not been possible to account for the Medicaid population in a similar fashion because we lack the requisite data on the extent of private insurance coverage among the medically indigent. Only the *net* addition of persons to the insured roll is of concern to us here.

U_t: We assume that the extra utilization of insured persons is directly proportional to the level of real benefits received, or

$$U_t = 1 + \frac{n B_t}{CP_t}, \qquad (2)$$

where B_t = average benefits per insured, in dollar terms. This is measured as private insurance benefits for 1948-65, and private insurance plus Medicare Part B benefits [59] for 1966-68.

n = increase in utilization ratio for each dollar of real benefits. The customary price index is the appropriate price deflator for benefits: to the extent services are covered by insurance, they are very likely to be paid for at their full customary price. Data for 1963 are used to determine the constant n, since this is the only year for which a direct calculation of U_t can be made; fortunately, the year falls in the second of our three periods of observation rather than at either end.

Utilization is measured not by the total number of visits, but rather by the value of services received.[3] There is much variation in the cost of different types of visits, and it seems reasonable that insurance coverage not only raises the total number of visits but also affects their average quality, shifting demand away from the less expensive outpatient visits to the more costly inpatient visits. Indeed, most policies offer little or no coverage for outpatient care. There would be a downward bias in our estimate of U_t if this fact were not taken into account.

The first step in computing a meaningful measure of relative utilization in 1963 is to distinguish the relevant classes of visits. The total utilization of physicians' services by the average insured (uninsured) person is arrived at by determining the number of visits he makes of each class and then weighting the different visits according to their relative value (i.e., customary fee) and summing over all classes. Of course, it is not necessary to know the absolute number of visits of each kind; it is sufficient to know the distribution of visits by class for one group, say the insured, and the insured/uninsured visit ratio applicable to each class of visit. The formula for determining the overall utilization ratio is thus:

$$U_t = \frac{\Sigma_i S_i R_i}{\Sigma_i S_i / U_{ti} R_i} \qquad (3)$$

where S_i = per cent of insured person's visits of class i; R_i = relative cost of a class i visit; and U_{ti} = relative number of class i visits by insured persons versus uninsured persons.

We distinguish 3 classes of visits: outpatient visits (O), hospital inpatient visits of a surgical variety (HS), and all other hospital inpatient visits (HM). The visit ratio for O

---

[2] The programs include Defense Department medical care (including military dependents), maternal and child health services, veterans' hospital medical care, workmen's compensation, public assistance, health insurance for the aged, temporary disability insurance, and medical vocational rehabilitation.

[3] We note that Feldstein chose the former method.

is obtained from the 1963-64 National Health Survey. Data on outpatient visits [56, pp. 13, 29] and surgical insurance status of the sample population [53, p. 3] are given for five income classes (j). Regressing per capita visits on the per cent of persons insured,

$$V_j = c + a\, INS_j + u_j\,, \tag{4}$$

gives us an estimate of the number of visits per uninsured ($c = 3.939$) and per insured ($c + a = 4.876$), implying a utilization ratio of 1.24 for class O visits. Its low value is not surprising, since surgical insurance policies (as indeed all physician insurance policies) generally do not reimburse expenses incurred for outpatient visits.

The Health Information Foundation-National Opinion Research Center survey reports six surgical procedures per 100 person-years for people with surgical and/or medical insurance, and three procedures per 100 person-years for those without either kind of insurance [3, p. 29]. The utilization ratio for HS is thus 2.0.

Lastly, we assume that the relative utilization of insured persons for HM visits is dependent upon the degree to which they are also covered by regular medical (RM) policies.[4] Specifically, those with RM will demonstrate the 2.0 utilization characteristic of surgically insured persons on surgical visits, while those without it will demonstrate the 1.24 rate characteristic of generally uncovered outpatient visits. Approximately 78 per cent of those with S also had RM in 1963,[5] so the visit ratio for HM in that year is estimated as $1.24\,(0.22) + 2.00\,(0.78) = 1.81$.

Total Charges, Total Visits, and Charge per Visit for Six Classes of Physician Visits, January 1968

	Total Charges (Millions)	Total Visits (Thous.)	Average Charge per Visit
All	$203.3	20,091	$10.12
Outpatient			
1. Home Visits	10.8	1,141	9.47
2. Office Visits	62.8	7,132	8.74
3. Outpatient Care	7.4	882	8.39
4. Nursing Home Care	12.3	2,696	4.56
Hospital Inpatient			
5. Surgical Inpatient	54.4	1,498	36.32
6. Other Inpatient	56.1	6,742	8.32

Source: [58].

---

[4] Recall that the definition of I_t, above, refers essentially to surgical insurance status (S).

[5] This assumes everyone with RM also had S.

Information regarding the distribution of total visits of insured persons and the customary charge for each class of visit is from [58], based upon a survey of Medicare enrollees with supplementary medical insurance coverage. As it happens, only surgical inpatient visits (7.4 per cent of the total) are priced markedly out of line with other types of visits. Inpatient visits of a nonsurgical nature (34.1 per cent) can therefore be considered together with outpatient visits (58.5 per cent) in our utilization formula, since apparently they do not entail any additional utilization of physicians' services. A weighted average of customary charges for these outpatient and inpatient nonsurgical visits is $7.99, as compared to $36.32 for the surgical inpatient visit; the relative cost of surgical visits is thus 4.55. The utilization ratio applicable to the combined O-HM visits is 1.42 (a weighted average of 1.24 and 1.81, the weights being the per cent of total visits in each class), as compared to 2.0 for the costlier surgical visits. The overall utilization rate is therefore computed as

$$U_{1963}$$

$$= \frac{0.074\,(4.55) + 0.926\,(1)}{(1/2)\,(0.074)\,(4.55) + (1/1.42)\,(0.926)\,(1)} = 1.55 \tag{5}$$

Insurance benefits per enrollee were $17.14 in 1963, and the customary fee index stood at 114.4, giving a "real" benefit figure of $14.98 in 1957-59 dollars. Substituting into (2), we solve for the constant n:

$$r = \frac{U_t - 1}{B_t/CP_t} = \frac{1.55 - 1}{14.98} = 0.037.$$

Each real dollar of insurance benefits raises the utilization of an insured person 3.7 per cent above that of an uninsured person. Since B_t and CP_t are known for all years, (2) can now be used to develop a U_t series:

$$U_t = 1 + 0.037\,\frac{B_t}{CP_t}.$$

k and K_t: The payments ratio for uninsured persons (k) is assumed to be constant. For insured persons it is allowed to vary with the fraction of their expenditures reimbursed; we assume they pay the full customary price to the extent they are covered, and at a rate (k^*) midway between k and 1 on their uninsured expenditures:[6]

$$k^* = (1 + k)/2. \tag{6}$$

---

[6] We have, rather arbitrarily, placed k^* midway between k and 1. The reasoning behind this is twofold: (1) Insured persons are concentrated among the middle- and upper-income groups.

(Footnote cont'd on page 50)

$k*$ is also assumed to be constant. We have not found it possible to directly compute either of these constants from data in published sources, but, as in the case of n, we can derive these constants indirectly, using the data for 1963. Since expenditures for each group are equal to utilization multiplied by the payments ratio, we may write

$$U_t = \frac{U_{It}}{U_{Nt}} = \frac{E_{It}/K_t}{E_{Nt}/k}$$

$$= \frac{b_t E_{It} + (1 - b_t) E_{It}/k*}{E_{Nt}/k} = \frac{k}{K_t} E_t , \qquad (7)$$

where

E_{It}, E_{Nt} = expenditures per insured, uninsured in year t;

b_t = fraction of insured person's expenditures reimbursed by insurance (and hence representing services paid for at their full value) in year t;

k = payments ratio of uninsured person;

$k*$ = payments ratio of insured persons on uninsured purchases;

K_t = average payments ratio of insured persons in year t;

E_t = E_{It}/E_{Nt} = expenditures ratio in year t.

Thus a knowledge of U_t, E_t, and b_t for any one year will allow us to solve for k, using the formula

$$\frac{U_t}{E_t} = k [b_t + (1 - b_t)/k*] = kb_t + \frac{2k (1 - b_t)}{1 + k} . \qquad (8)$$

(Footnote cont'd from page 49)

Relative income of a patient is probably as important as insurance status in determining the size of the price discount he will be granted and the extent to which he pays his bills. (2) When the physician is aware that his patient possesses insurance, he will probably be less inclined to grant price discounts even though he realizes that insurance coverage is rarely comprehensive. Since the insured party need not pay at all for one portion of the services received, the physician may insist that he pay relatively more than uninsured persons for nonreimbursed services, though not necessarily that he pay for their full value.

The expenditures ratio for 1963 is derived from the NHS survey in the same fashion as is the outpatient visit utilization ratio.[7] Regressing per capita expenditures [55, pp. 7 and 29] on per cent with surgical insurance [56, p. 3] for five income classes,

$$E_j = c + a\ INS_j + u_j, \qquad (9)$$

we estimate E_{1963} to be $(c + a)/c$, or 2.08.

The value of b_t is readily computed as the ratio of total insurance benefits to total expenditures of insured persons. Benefits in 1963 accounted for 36.0 per cent of private expenditures ($2,311 million/$6,416 million).[8] 72.2 per cent of the population was insured in 1963, and their share of private expenditures was $E_{It} I_t/(E_{It} I_t + E_{Nt} N_t)$.

$$\frac{E_{It}I_t}{E_{Nt}N_t} = 2.08 \cdot \frac{72.2\%}{27.8\%} = \frac{150.2\%}{27.8\%} \qquad (10)$$

$$\frac{E_{It}I_t}{E_{It}I_t + E_{Nt}N_t} = \frac{150.2\%}{177.8\%} = 84.4\% \qquad (11)$$

$$b_t = \frac{\text{total benefits}}{E_{It}I_t} = \frac{36.0\%}{84.4\%} = 42.7\% \text{ in } 1963 \qquad (12)$$

For other years, the expenditures ratio ($E_t = E_{It}/E_{Nt}$) which figures in (10) is unknown and so b_t must be computed in a different fashion. We know that total expenditures equals expenditures of insured persons plus expenditures of uninsured persons:

$$EXPS_t = E_{It}I_t + E_{Nt} N_t. \qquad (13)$$

E_{It} equals the value of services received by the average insured person times the payments ratio K_t; an equivalent formulation is benefits (the value of insured services) per insured plus the value of uncompensated services multiplied by their payments ratio $k*$:

$$E_{It} = K_t U_{It} = K_t U_t U_{Nt} = \frac{K_t U_t E_{Nt}}{k}$$

$$= B_t + k* \left[\frac{U_t E_{Nt}}{k} - B_t \right] . \qquad (14)$$

---

[7] The survey questionnaire defines expenditures as all doctor's bills paid (or to be paid) by the person himself (or his family or friends) and any part paid by insurance, whether paid directly to the doctor or to the person himself.

[8] Only private expenditures should be considered in this context because E_t is derived from data on private expenditures.

Substituting (14) into (13) and solving, we have

$$E_{Nt} = \frac{EXPS_t - I_t\, B_t\,(1-k^*)}{N_t + I_t\,(k^*/k)\,U_t} \tag{15}$$

and

$$E_{It} = \frac{EXPS_t - E_{Nt}\,N_t}{I_t}. \tag{16}$$

We then solve (12) for b_t in years other than 1963 by using dollar figures for benefits and for expenditures of the insured from (16) rather than by using percentages, as in (10) through (12). The appropriate expenditures concept for this purpose is private expenditures (direct consumer expenditures plus private insurance benefits) plus Medicare benefits.

Substituting the 1963 value for b_t into (8), we have $\frac{1.55}{2.08} = 0.427\,k + \frac{1.146\,k}{1+k}$. Solving, we have the payments ratio of uninsured persons: $k = 0.67$. Substituting into (6) and (7), we have a formula for computing the annual payments ratio of insured persons,

$$k^* = 0.835$$

$$K_t = \frac{1}{b_t + (1=b_t)/k^*} = \frac{0.835}{1 - 0.165\,b_t}$$

Having solved for all constants, we proceed as follows to derive the average price series:

1. B_t = Benefits per insured (total benefits$_t \div I_t$);

2. $U_t = 1 + 0.037\dfrac{B_t}{CP_t}$;

3. $E_{Nt} = \dfrac{EXPS_t - \text{total benefits}_t\,(1-0.835)}{N_t + I_t\dfrac{0.835}{0.67}U_t}$;

4. $E_{it} = \dfrac{EXPS_t - N_t\,E_{Nt}}{I_t}$;

5. $b_t = \dfrac{B_t}{E_{it}}$;

6. $K_t = \dfrac{0.835}{1 - 0.165\,b_t}$;

7. $AP_t = \dfrac{U_t\,I_t\,K_t + N_t\,(0.67)}{U_t\,I_t + N_t} \cdot CP_t$.

Appendix C. Cross Section: Sources and Methods

EXP:

1966 gross annual business receipts of physicians in self-employment practice [61, pp. 55-73; 142-56]. This material was originally published in [33, pp. 96-98]. We have restricted our sample to the thirty-three states for which data are available on both sole proprietorships and partnerships. Excluded from the sample are Alaska, Delaware, District of Columbia, Hawaii, Idaho, Maine, Massachusetts, Montana, Nevada, New Hampshire, New Mexico, North Dakota, Rhode Island, South Dakota, Utah, Vermont, West Virginia, and Wyoming.

Q:

Number of general practitioner (G. P.) outpatient visits or their equivalent.

AP:

Average price of a G. P. outpatient visit equivalent. Q and AP are implicitly defined by the identity

$$EXP \equiv Q \cdot AP. \tag{1}$$

We estimate Q for each state directly, employing our knowledge of outpatient visits, inpatient visits, and the extent of physician specialization, and then obtain AP from (1).

Total outpatient visit equivalents are equivalent to the sum of such visits by G. P.'s and such visits by specialists.

$$V = V_g G + V_s S = V_g (G + bS), \tag{2}$$

and total expenditures can similarly be decomposed into expenditures for G. P.'s and expenditures for specialists,

$$EXP = P_g V_g G + P_s V_s S = P_g V_g (G + abS), \tag{3}$$

where P_g, P_s = average price per G. P., specialist outpatient visit equivalent; V_g, V_s = number of outpatient visit equivalents per G.P., specialist; G, S = number of G. P.'s, specialists; $P_s/P_g = a$, $V_s/V_g = b$. P_g is equivalent to AP, and thus:

$$Q = V_g (G + abS). \tag{4}$$

The number of outpatient visit equivalents, V, is defined by

$$V = O + wH, \tag{5}$$

where O = home and office visits; H = hospital inpatient visits; and w = outpatient visit equivalents per inpatient visit.

After appropriate substitutions, we have

$$Q = \frac{(O + wH)(G + abS)}{G + bS} \tag{6}$$

and

$$AP = EXP/Q. \tag{7}$$

According to (6), the quantity of physicians' services in a state equals the number of outpatient visit equivalents multiplied by a factor indicating the number of G. P. equivalent visits in the average physician visit. Sources for the right-hand side terms in (6) are described below.

O:

The National Center for Health Statistics provides data on number of home and office visits per capita for the four census regions in 1966-67 [57] and for the nine divisions in 1957-59 [52]. Home and office visits together accounted for 75 per cent of the total physician visits reported in the 1966-67 National Health Survey. We exclude visits in hospital outpatient clinics and emergency rooms (10 per cent) because these are performed by hospital physicians, not private practitioners. Also excluded are telephone visits (10 per cent), which are generally free of charge and represent much less utilization than in-person visits. The additional 5 per cent of visits occurred in company and industry health units, other places, or sites unknown.

We assume an intraregion distribution of per capita visits in 1966-67 comparable to the distribution that prevailed in the earlier period:

$$1957\text{-}59:\ O_1^* = O_1^* a W_{1a} + O_1^* b W_{1b} + \ \ldots. \tag{8}$$

$$1966\text{-}67:\ O_2^* = \frac{(O_1^* a)}{O_1^*} O_2^* W_{2a} +$$

$$\frac{(O_1^* b)}{O_1^*} O_2^* W_{2b} + \ldots, \tag{9}$$

where

$O^*_{i(j)}$ = per capita home and office visits for this region at time i (in division j).

W_{ij} = per cent of region's population residing in division j at time i.

In this way we can estimate 1966-67 per capita home and office visits for each of the divisions in a region by the term $(O^*_{1j}) \cdot (O^*_2)/O^*_1$. We then impute the same figure to each state in the division.

H:

We assume one hospital visit by a private practice physician for each day of stay in a nonfederal, short-term hospital. 1966 days of stay, the product of admissions and average length of stay, are known for each state [25, Aug. 1, 1967]. Our assumption is supported by survey data which indicate that the median number of hospital visits by self-employed physicians was 22 per week in 1966, and that the median number of weeks worked per year was 48 (in 1968) [30]. If physicians in these thirty-three states conformed to the national medians, they would have made 177 million hospital visits; in fact, the number of patient days in these states was quite close to this—185 million.

w:

The 1968 national ratio of average charge for a hospital inpatient visit relative to a home or office visit, or 1.71. Data apply to the Medicare population [58].

G, S:

Applies to physicians in private practice in 1966 [2, 1967].

a:

National ratio of specialists' average gross receipts per visit (AGR) to those of general practitioners. We assume that this ratio is the same for total visits (to which the data apply) as for outpatient visit equivalents. The AGR for G. P.'s was $5.48, computed from survey data for solo practitioners on 1966 median annual gross income from self-employment practice and number of annual visits (median weeks per year times median visits per week). Computation was made for each kind of practitioner, with G. P.'s and selected kinds of specialists together accounting for 80 per cent of self-employed solo physicians. A weighted average for the specialists was $10.55. Thus, a = 1.93, assumed constant for all states [30].

b:

1966 median number of weekly visits per specialist (a weighted average of all kinds of specialists) relative to median number of weekly visits per G. P., or 0.625, assumed constant for all states [30]. Again, we assume this ratio to be the same for total visits (to which the data apply) as for outpatient visit equivalents.

MD:

Number of nonfederal physicians active in "solo, partnership, group, and other practice." MD = G + S. The series excludes nonfederal physicians primarily engaged in teaching, research, industry, public health, or hospital-based practice.

BEN:

1966 private insurance benefits for physicians' services. Because data are not published on the type of health insurance benefits paid in each state, we estimate BEN from data on total health insurance benefit payments for a state (this includes hospital expense and disability income payments as well as physician expense) and on the number of state residents protected by the various kinds of policies (published only for hospital, surgical, and regular medical policies).

We assume first that hospital expense and physician expense benefits together constituted 89 per cent of the benefit total, since this is the ratio that prevailed nationally in that year. Then we separate out the physician expense benefits by assuming that the national ratio of hospital benefits per hospital insured to physician benefits per surgically insured (1.76) prevailed in each state. The data are from [23, 1967 and 1968]. Thus,

(1) $HIB = HOS + BEN + DI$;

(2) $0.89\, HIB \approx HOS + BEN$;

(3) $BEN + HOS = bB + hH \approx b\,(B + 1.76H)$;

(4) $BEN = bB \approx \dfrac{.89\, HIB\,(B)}{B + 1.76H}$,

where HIB = total health insurance benefits, 1966; HOS, BEN, DI = hospital expense, physician expense, and disability income benefit payments, 1966; h, b = hospital, physician benefits per person with hospital, physician expense protection; H, B = number of persons with hospital, physician expense protection. B, the number of persons with *any* physician insurance (surgical, regular medical, or major medical), is not precisely known, owing to an undetermined number of policyholders with two or more forms of coverage. The number of surgically insured persons serves as a very good proxy for B (see Appendix B). H and B are only available for the population under age sixty-five, but this should not bias the results, since only their ratio is of consequence.

PRM/BEN:

Ratio of all health insurance premiums to all health insurance benefits [23, 1968].

INC*:

1966 per capita disposable personal income [49, p. 29].

MED SCLS:

1966 [1, Nov. 21, 1966].

BEDS:

Beds in nonfederal, short-term general and other special hospitals, as of Mar. 1, 1967 [2]; from statistics collected by American Hospital Association.

UNION:

1966 labor union members [47, 1969, p. 236].

POPULATION:

July 1, 1966 civilian resident population [44].

The following variables also appeared in the preliminary large-scale version of our model:

DTH RT:

Average of 1965, 1966, and 1967 death rate per 1,000 residents [47, 1968, p. 56 and 1969, p. 56].

ΔINC*:

1966 INC* minus 1960 INC* [49, p. 29].

INF MRT:

1966. Deaths of infants under one year old, exclusive of fetal deaths, per 1,000 live births. A weighted average of published series for white and nonwhite births [47, 1968].

EDUC:

Median years of school completed by persons twenty-five years old and over [43, pp. 1-20, Table 12].

%URB:

1960. Per cent of total population classified as urban [43, p. xvi].

AGED:

Persons sixty-five years and over, July 1, 1966 [44], as per cent of population.

BRTH RT:

1966 live births, white plus nonwhite, per 1,000 persons [47, 1968, p. 55].

%BLK:

1960 [47, 1969, p. 27].

S&L GOV:

Fiscal 1967 state and local government expenditures for hospitals and "other health" [42, Table 18 of each state volume].

TEMP:

[47, 1969, p. 174] lists one average annual figure for all but fourteen states in our sample (California, Florida, Illinois, Michigan, Missouri, New York, North Carolina, Ohio, Pennsylvania, Tennessee, Texas, Virginia, Washington). For these states, characterized by greater geographic variation in temperature and more widely dispersed populations, temperatures are given for two or three major cities. We have used a weighted average of the city figures (with the cities' populations as weights) as the basis for our TEMP variable in these cases.

%SPEC:

Specialists active in nonfederal, "solo, partnership, group, and other practice," as a per cent of MD [2, 1967].

HOSP MD:

Nonfederal, hospital-based physicians in 1966 [2, 1967].

%PART:

Number of physicians filing partnership business income tax returns for medical practice in 1966 as a per cent of total number of physicians so filing (sole proprietors plus partners) [61 or 33].

MD ORIG:

The sum of the number of first-year medical students originating from a state in each of six selected years (chosen so as to constitute a fairly representative sample of the 1966 physician stock). In the published data, state of origin is variously denoted as "birthplace" (1936, 1941), "residence" (1947, 1953, 1957), and "geographic source" (1961). The data for 1936 and 1941 apply to all medical students and hence describe the state of origin of entering students in the years 1933-36 and 1938-41, respectively; so as not to give undue weight to these years, only one-fourth of this figure enters the computation of MD ORIG [1, various issues].

Table C-1

Expenditures, Insurance, and Price, 1966

State	Total Expenditures (Thousands)	Physician Insurance Benefits per Capita (BEN*)	Per Cent of Persons with Surgical Insurance	Average Price (AP)	Net Price (NP)
Alabama	$110,519	$10.70	64.0	$4.96	$3.28
Arizona	83,252	12.40	47.4	7.22	5.52
Arkansas	57,612	8.25	45.9	4.84	3.49
California	1,265,801	17.20	67.7	8.31	6.23
Colorado	118,863	19.00	69.5	7.52	5.22
Connecticut	146,044	19.80	77.4	7.54	4.62
Florida	238,515	11.40	62.3	5.19	3.76
Georgia	148,515	11.10	74.5	4.87	3.29
Illinois	497,902	18.50	78.0	5.96	3.59
Indiana	200,540	17.30	75.8	5.86	3.37
Iowa	91,801	14.30	71.7	4.53	2.58
Kansas	98,479	13.10	59.9	5.78	4.05
Kentucky	118,176	10.10	57.0	5.94	4.35
Louisiana	158,431	8.86	49.5	6.06	4.85
Maryland	158,908	12.60	54.7	6.00	4.33
Michigan	340,574	24.10	79.6	5.23	2.11
Minnesota	125,355	16.00	71.3	4.22	2.31

(continued)

Table C-1 (concluded)

State	Total Expenditures (Thousands)	Physician Insurance Benefits per Capita (BEN*)	Per Cent of Persons with Surgical Insurance	Average Price (AP)	Net Price (NP)
Mississippi	$65,498	$8.17	47.1	$5.03	$3.58
Missouri	171,546	15.50	69.4	4.62	2.73
Nebraska	61,456	12.40	67.8	5.83	4.14
New Jersey	317,426	16.60	66.6	5.85	3.76
New York	895,435	22.30	86.2	5.55	3.04
North Carolina	161,411	9.72	68.6	4.54	3.21
Ohio	477,388	18.80	78.9	6.15	3.64
Oklahoma	85,159	11.30	69.4	5.11	3.46
Oregon	125,217	12.80	61.1	7.89	6.31
Pennsylvania	427,291	17.50	76.9	4.35	2.29
South Carolina	66,278	8.70	67.7	3.92	2.63
Tennessee	134,408	12.90	68.3	4.97	3.14
Texas	423,597	12.70	61.5	5.70	3.91
Virginia	160,820	12.00	56.4	5.15	3.50
Washington	138,211	16.20	71.5	6.00	3.90
Wisconsin	163,130	18.00	77.5	4.99	2.70

Table C-2

Physicians by Type of Practice, 1966

State	Physicians in Private Practice	Specialists in Private Practice
Alabama	2,190	1,321
Arizona	1,491	1,000
Arkansas	1,310	621
California	24,465	16,895

(continued)

Table C-2 (concluded)

State	Physicians in Private Practice	Specialists in Private Practice
Colorado	2,207	1,558
Connecticut	3,412	2,571
Florida	5,353	3,910
Georgia	3,084	2,048
Illinois	9,979	6,164
Indiana	3,896	2,122
Iowa	2,093	1,023
Kansas	1,729	952
Kentucky	2,237	1,279
Louisiana	2,804	1,904
Maryland	3,211	2,279
Michigan	6,603	4,469
Minnesota	3,342	2,044
Mississippi	1,385	702
Missouri	3,577	2,446
Nebraska	1,246	649
New Jersey	6,905	4,730
New York	24,292	17,347
North Carolina	3,450	2,225
Ohio	9,135	5,865
Oklahoma	1,873	1,101
Oregon	2,002	1,320
Pennsylvania	11,249	7,052
South Carolina	1,605	891
Tennessee	2,986	1,986
Texas	8,679	5,471
Virginia	3,486	2,277
Washington	3,162	2,021
Wisconsin	3,611	2,217

Table C-3

Weighted, Logarithmic Correlation Matrix, 1966

(N=33 states)

	EXP*	Q*	AP	NP	BEN*	MD*	EXP/MD	Q/MD	DTH RT	INF MRT	INC*	MED SCLS[a]
Q*	.55											
AP	.91	.15										
NP	.71	-.07	.88									
BEN*	.50	.70	.24	-.21								
MD*	.83	.79	.59	.38	.64							
EXP/MD	.27	-.43	.54	.57	-.26	-.31						
Q/MD	-.84	-.52	-.74	-.57	-.49	-.93	.18					
DTH RT	-.27	.29	-.47	-.53	.25	.01	-.49	.15				
INF MRT	-.52	-.58	-.33	-.05	-.67	-.58	.11	.46	-.12			
INC*	.73	.73	.49	.14	.86	.79	-.12	-.67	.15	-.74		
MED SCLS[a]	.44	.72	.16	-.01	.55	.73	-.52	-.60	.25	-.24	.51	
UNION*	.50	.64	.27	-.12	.87	.59	-.17	-.45	.41	-.69	.82	.46
BEDS*	-.01	.54	-.29	-.39	.36	.23	-.43	-.00	.60	-.36	.25	.39
PRM/BEN	-.59	-.55	-.42	-.08	-.71	-.63	.07	.55	.06	.46	-.64	-.44
%SPEC[a]	.59	.59	.37	.23	.41	.63	-.14	-.54	-.15	-.14	.45	.43
ΔINC*	.36	.42	.21	-.12	.68	.40	-.08	-.31	.16	-.61	.78	.25
EDUC	.78	.54	.66	.41	.60	.70	.13	-.66	-.12	-.73	.77	.23
%AGED[a]	-.03	.34	-.21	-.23	.20	.18	-.37	-.05	.77	-.36	.22	.13
%BLK[a]	-.53	-.55	-.35	-.07	-.69	-.56	.07	.47	-.18	.89	-.72	-.22
%PART[a]	-.16	-.21	-.08	-.04	-.21	-.30	.26	.30	-.30	-.03	-.28	-.40
BRTH RT	-.20	-.51	.03	.09	-.34	-.42	.41	.29	-.60	.50	-.37	-.34
MD ORIG*	-.40	.10	-.53	-.58	.17	-.08	-.55	.18	.61	-.10	-.02	.22
S&L GOV*	.44	.55	.24	.07	.45	.61	-.30	-.52	.05	-.19	.46	.61
HOSP MD*	.43	.79	.11	-.16	.72	.69	-.46	-.49	.27	-.46	.68	.68
TEMP	-.07	-.40	.13	.43	-.68	-.21	.25	.05	-.45	.64	-.55	-.13
%URB[a]	.77	.70	.55	.27	.73	.82	-.11	-.74	.01	-.51	.85	.57

[a]Linear variable.

TABLE C-3 (Concluded)

UNION*	BEDS*	PRM/BEN	%SPEC[a]	ΔINC*	EDUC	%AGED[a]	%BLK[a]	%PART[a]	BRTH RT	MD ORIG*	S&L GOV*	HOSP MD*	TEMP
.37													
-.68	-.10												
.30	-.09	-.55											
.65	.19	-.28	.11										
.51	.13	-.51	.29	.52									
.27	.61	.13	-.10	.16	.26								
-.68	-.43	.44	-.12	-.53	-.75	-.46							
-.23	.12	.26	-.36	-.02	-.02	-.10	.03						
-.38	-.46	.12	-.09	-.13	-.35	-.71	.56	.33					
.20	.60	.04	-.33	.07	-.30	.30	-.05	-.03	-.29				
.35	.17	-.32	.53	.38	.29	.11	-.11	.02	-.06	.04			
.67	.43	-.63	.68	.48	.33	.16	-.40	-.34	-.32	.25	.56		
-.72	-.54	.30	.06	-.63	-.25	-.30	.62	-.14	.31	-.48	-.11	-.49	
.66	.12	-.73	.64	.42	.70	.12	-.54	-.41	-.27	-.17	.46	.62	-.17

BIBLIOGRAPHY

1. American Medical Association. *Journal of the American Medical Association.* Annual education issue: Aug. 15, 1937; Aug. 28, 1942; Sept. 4, 1948; Sept. 1, 1954; Nov. 15, 1958; Nov. 17, 1962; Nov. 21, 1966.

2. American Medical Association, Dept. of Survey Research. *Distribution of Physicians, Hospitals, and Hospital Beds in the U.S.: Regional, State, County, Metropolitan Area.* Chicago (annually since 1963).

3. Andersen, Ronald, and Anderson, Odin W. *A Decade of Health Services: Social Survey Trends in Use and Expenditure.* Chicago: University of Chicago Press, 1967.

4. Andersen, Ronald, and Benham, Lee. "Factors Affecting the Relationship Between Family Income and Medical Care Consumption." In Herbert Klarman, ed., *Empirical Studies in Health Economics.* Baltimore: Johns Hopkins Press, 1970, pp. 73-95.

5. Auster, Richard; Leveson, Irving; and Sarachek, Deborah. "The Production of Health, an Exploratory Study." In Victor R. Fuchs, ed., *Essays in the Economics of Health and Medical Care.* New York: NBER, 1972.

6. Barnes, Allan C. "The Missing Evidence." *Perspectives in Biology and Medicine* (Autumn 1970).

7. Benham, L.; Maurizi, A.; and Reder, M. W. "Migration, Location, and Remuneration of Medical Personnel: Physicians and Dentists." *Review of Economics and Statistics* 50 (August 1968): 332-47.

8. Brewster, Agnes. "Voluntary Health Insurance and Private Medical Care Expenditures, 1948-59." *Social Security Bulletin* 23 (December 1960).

9. Chiswick, Barry R., and Mincer, Jacob. "Time Series Changes in Personal Income Inequality in the United States from 1939, with Projections to 1985." *Journal of Political Economy* 80 (May/June 1972 supplement): 534-66.

10. Cooper, Barbara S. "National Health Expenditures, 1929-67." U.S. Dept. of Health, Education, and Welfare, Social Security Administration, Office of Research and Statistics. *Research and Statistics Note,* No. 16 (Sept. 29, 1969).

11. Cooper, Barbara S. "National Health Expenditures, Fiscal Years 1929-69 and Calendar Years 1929-68." *Research and Statistics Note,* No. 18 (Nov. 7, 1969).

12. Cooper, Barbara S. and McGee, Mary. *Compendium of National Health Expenditures Data.* U.S. Dept. of Health, Education, and Welfare, Social Security Administration, Office of Research and Statistics, 1971. (In process.)

13. Costello, P. M. "Technological Progress in the Ethical Drug Industry." In *Competitive Problems in the Drug Industry,* Hearings before the Subcommittee on Monopoly of the Select Committee of Small Business, United States Senate, 90th Congress, 1st and 2nd sessions of Present Status of Competition in the Pharmaceutical Industry, Part V, 1968.

14. *Economic Report of the President.* Washington, D.C.: February 1970.

15. Fein, Rashi. *The Doctor Shortage: An Economic Diagnosis.* Washington, D.C.: Brookings Institution, 1967.

16. Feldstein, Martin S. "The Rising Price of Physicians' Services." *The Review of Economics and Statistics* 52 (May 1970); 121-33.

17. Feldstein, Paul J. "The Demand for Medical Care." In *Commission on the Cost of Medical Care, General Report,* Vol. I. Chicago: American Medical Association, 1964, pp. 57-76.

18. Fuchs, Victor R. *The Service Economy.* New York: NBER, 1968.

19. Fuchs, Victor R. "Some Economic Aspects of Mortality in the United States." New York: NBER, 1966. Mimeo.

20. Fuchs, Victor, and Grossman, Michael. "The Correlation Between Health and Schooling." New York: NBER, 1970. Mimeo.

21. Ginzberg, Eli. *Men, Money, and Medicine.* New York: Columbia University Press, 1969.

22. Grossman, Michael. *The Demand for Health: A Theoretical and Empirical Investigation.* New York: NBER, 1972.

23. Health Insurance Institute. *Source Book of Health Insurance Data.* New York (annually).

24. Holen, Arlene S. "Effects of Professional Licensing Arrangements on Interstate Labor Mobility and Resource Allocation." *The Journal of Political Economy* 73 (October 1965): 492-98.

25. *Hospitals: Journal of the American Hospital Association.* Guide Issue, Part 2 (annually).

26. Kessel, Reuben A. "Price Discrimination in Medicine." *Journal of Law and Economics* 1 (October 1958).

27. Klarman, Herbert. "Economic Aspects of Projecting Requirements for Health Manpower." *Journal of Human Resources* 4 (Summer 1969): 360-76.

28. Klarman, Herbert E.; Rice, Dorothy P.; Cooper, Barbara S.; and Stettler, Louis H. III. "Sources of Increase in Expenditures for Selected Health Services, 1929-69." U.S. Dept. of Health, Education, and Welfare, Social Security Administration, Office of Research and Statistics, Staff Paper No. 4 (April 1970).

29. *Medical Economics,* bi-weekly.

30. *Medical Economics.* Feb. 6, 1967, April 1, 1968, and Dec. 8, 1969.

31. Peterson, Paul Q., and Pennell, Maryland Y. *Health Manpower Source Book: Section 14, Medical Specialists.* U.S. Dept. of Health, Education, and Welfare, Public Health Service Publication No. 263. Washington, D.C.: 1962.

32. *Population and Vital Statistics Report of the United Nations.* Statistical Papers Series A, Vol. 22, No. 2. New York: 1970.

33. Reed, Louis S. *Studies of the Incomes of Physicians and Dentists.* U.S. Dept. of Health, Education, and Welfare, Social Security Administration, Office of Research and Statistics. SS Pub. 69-19 (3-69), December 1968.

34. Reed, Louis S., and Carr, Willine. *The Benefit Structure of Private Insurance.* U.S. Dept. of Health, Education, and Welfare, Social Security Administration, Office of Research and Statistics, Research Report No. 32, 1970.

35. Reed, Louis S., and Hanft, Ruth S. "National Health Expenditures, 1950-64." *Social Security Bulletin* 29 (January 1966): 18-19.

36. Rice, Dorothy P., and Cooper, Barbara S. "National Health Expenditures, 1929-68." *Social Security Bulletin* 33, No. 1 (January 1970).

37. Rimlinger, G. V., and Steele, H. B. "Income Opportunities and Physician Location Trends in the United States." *Western Economic Journal* (Spring 1965): 182-94.

38. Schultz, T. P. "Secular Trends and Cyclical Behavior of Income Distribution in the United States, 1944-1965." In Lee Soltow, ed., *Six Papers on the Size Distribution of Wealth and Income.* New York: NBER, 1969.

39. Schwartzman, David. "The Growth of Sales Per Man-Hour in Retail Trade, 1929-1963." In V. R. Fuchs, ed., *Production and Productivity in the Service Industries.* New York: NBER, 1969, pp. 223-25.

40. Silver, Morris. "An Economic Analysis of Variations in Medical Expenses and Work Loss Rates." In Victor R. Fuchs, ed., *Essays in the Economics of Health and Medical Care.* New York: NBER, 1972.

41. Sloan, Frank A. *Economic Models of Physician Supply.* Ph.D. dissertation, Harvard University, 1970.

42. U.S. Dept. of Commerce, Bureau of the Census. *1967 Census of Governments, State Reports,* V. 7.

43. U.S. Dept. of Commerce, Bureau of the Census. *Census of Population,* Vol. 1, Part A, 1960.

44. U.S. Dept. of Commerce, Bureau of the Census. *Current Population Reports* P-25, No. 380 (November 24, 1967).

45. U.S. Dept. of Commerce, Bureau of the Census. *Current Population Reports* P-25, No. 430 (August 29, 1969).

46. U.S. Dept. of Commerce, Bureau of the Census. *Historical Statistics of the U.S., Colonial Times to 1957,* and *Historical Statistics of the U.S., Continuation to 1962 and Revisions.* Washington, D.C.: 1960 and 1965, respectively.

47. U.S. Dept. of Commerce, Bureau of the Census. *Statistical Abstract of the United States* (annually).

48. U.S. Dept. of Commerce, Office of Business Economics. *The National Income and Product Accounts of the United States, 1929-65, Statistical Tables.* Washington, D.C.: 1966.

49. U.S. Dept. of Commerce, Office of Business Economics. *Survey of Current Business* 49, No. 4 (April 1969).

50. U.S. Dept. of Commerce, Office of Business Economics. *Survey of Current Business* 49, No. 7 (July 1969).

51. U.S. Dept. of Health, Education, and Welfare. *Fluoridation Census 1969.* Washington, D.C.: 1970.

52. U.S. Dept. of Health, Education, and Welfare, Public Health Service. "Selected Health Characteristics by Area, Geographic Divisions and Large Metropolitan Areas, United States, July 1957-June 1959. *Health Statistics from the National Health Survey,* Series C, No. 6 (March 1961).

53. U.S. Dept. of Health, Education, and Welfare, Public Health Service, National Center for Health Statistics. "Health Insurance Coverage, United States, July 1962-June 1963." *Vital and Health Statistics,* Series 10, No. 11 (1964).

54. U.S. Dept. of Health, Education, and Welfare, Public Health Service, National Center for Health Statistics. "Health Insurance. Type of Insuring Organization and Multiple Coverage, United States, July 1962-June 1963." *Vital and Health Statistics,* Series 10, No. 16 (1965).

55. U.S. Dept. of Health, Education, and Welfare, Public Health Service, National Center for Health Statistics. "Personal Health Expenses: Per Capita Annual Expenses, United States, July-December 1962." *Vital and Health Statistics,* Series 10, No. 27 (1966).

56. U.S. Dept. of Health, Education, and Welfare, Public Health Service, National Center for Health Statistics. "Volume of Physician Visits by Place of Visit and Type of Service, United States, July 1963-June 1964." *Vital and Health Statistics,* Series 10, No. 18 (1965).

57. U.S. Dept. of Health, Education, and Welfare, Public Health Service, National Center for Health Statistics. "Volume of Physician Visits, United States, July 1966-June 1967." *Vital and Health Statistics,* Series 10, No. 49 (November 1968).

58. U.S. Dept. of Health, Education, and Welfare, Social Security Administration, Office of Research and Statistics. "Current Medicare Survey Report." *Health Insurance Statistics* CMS-12 (January 27, 1970).

59. U.S. Dept. of Health, Education, and Welfare, Social Security Administration, Office of Research and Statistics. *Health Insurance Statistics* HI-11 (January 31, 1969), and HI-17 (April 15, 1970).

60. U.S. Dept. of Labor, Bureau of Labor Statistics. *The Consumer Price Index.* (December of each year.)

61. U.S. Dept. of Treasury, Internal Revenue Service. *Statistics of Income 1966: Business Income Tax Returns.* Washington, D.C.: 1969.

☆ U. S. GOVERNMENT PRINTING OFFICE : 1973 O - 492-589